Full Moon
Possible Side Effects!

By Jim Allen, EdD, RRT

&

(Your name)

Full Moon, Possible Side Effects! is a surreal look at the idiosyncratic world of healthcare. Chaos, insanity, bedlam, and a daily dose of a "perpetual full moon" creates an unstable concoction . When all those elements are aligned, Murphy's Law kicks in!

Full Moon, Possible Side Effects! is a collection of cartoons from the comics Full Moon and Full Moon Over Meshugga G.

The comics include the author's captions, but you might see something completely different. Under each comic is an area to add your captions. Interact with the comics and expand them with your own insights. Don't forget to add your name as the co-author.

Post them on the bulletin board for others to critique or add their own captions.

Full Moon Comics
FullMoonComics.com

Full Moon Comics
FullMoonComics.com

Dedicated to all healthcare professionals.

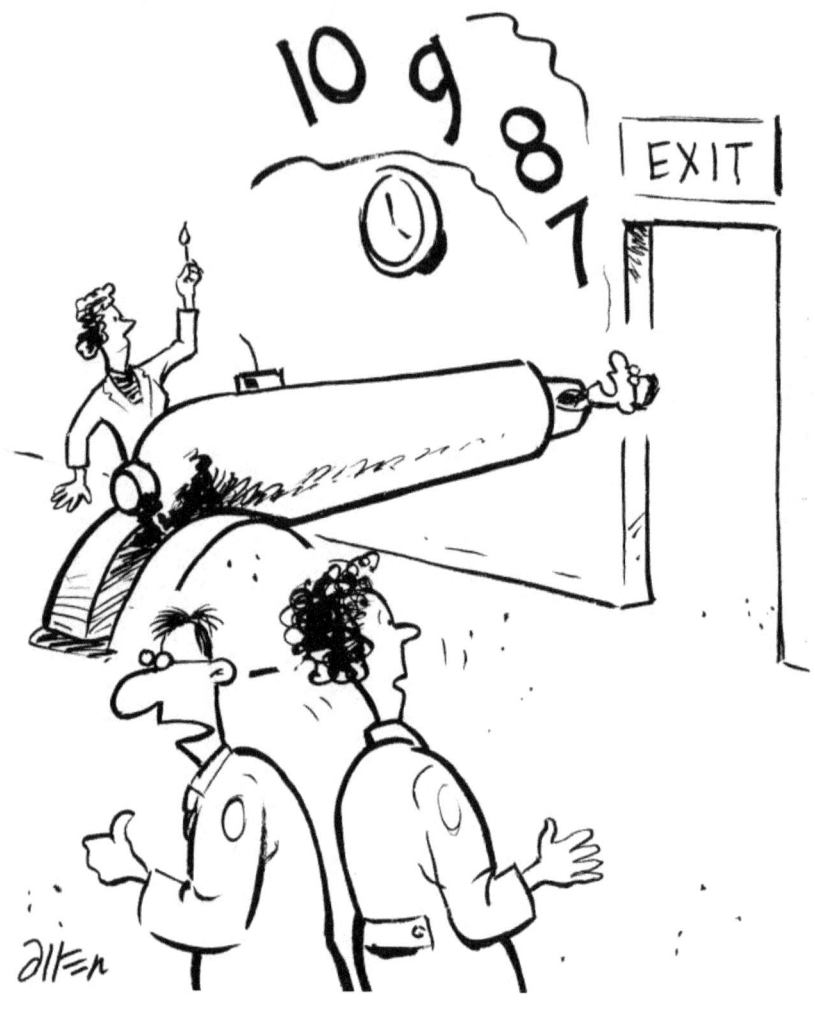

He does that at quitting time every day!

Enter your caption:

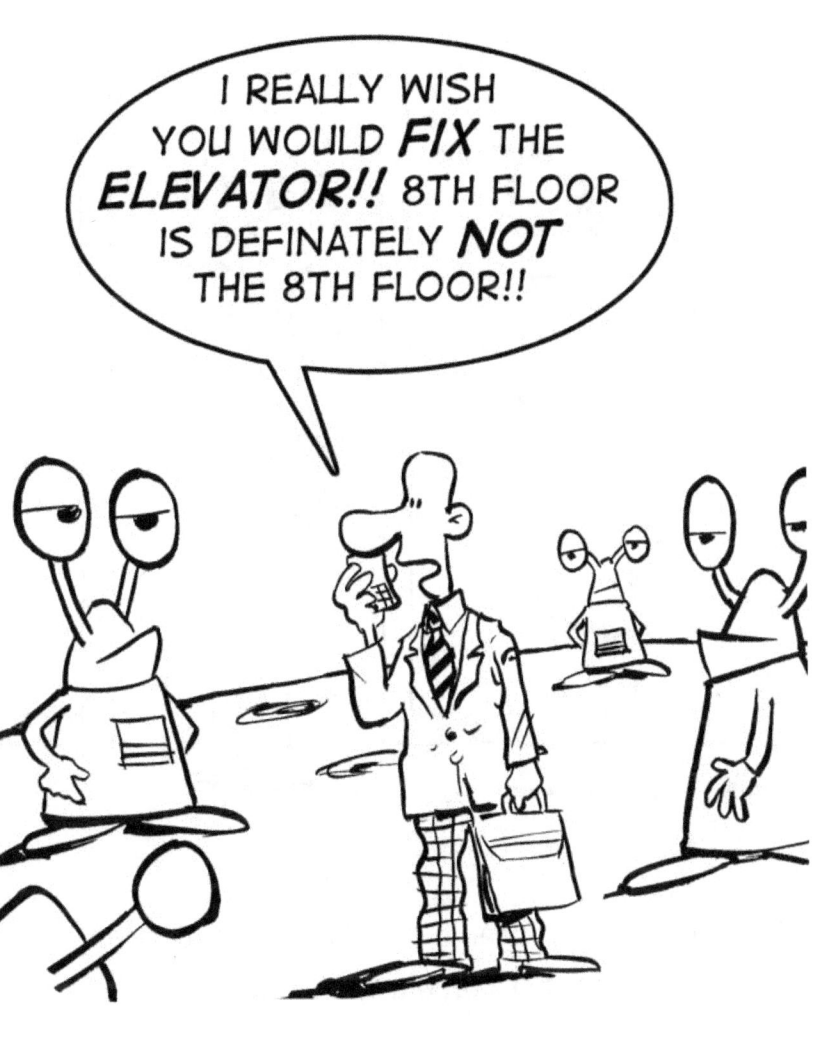

Enter your caption:

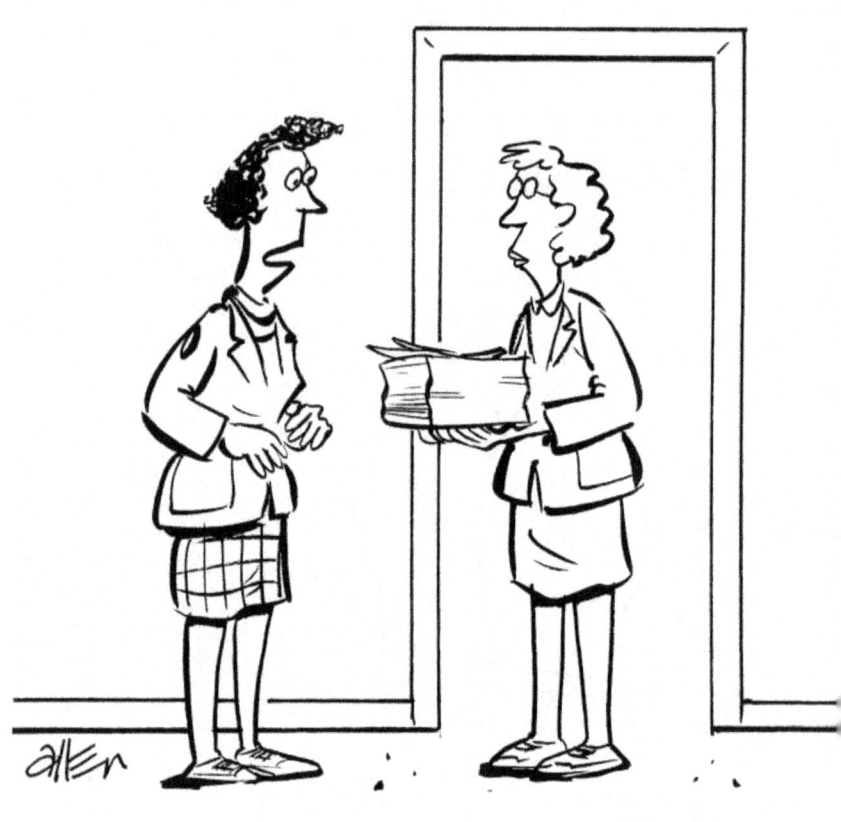

Just what do you mean by the "feng-shui deficiencies"
hit us hard on our last inspection?

Enter your caption:

_____

_____

_____

_____

_____

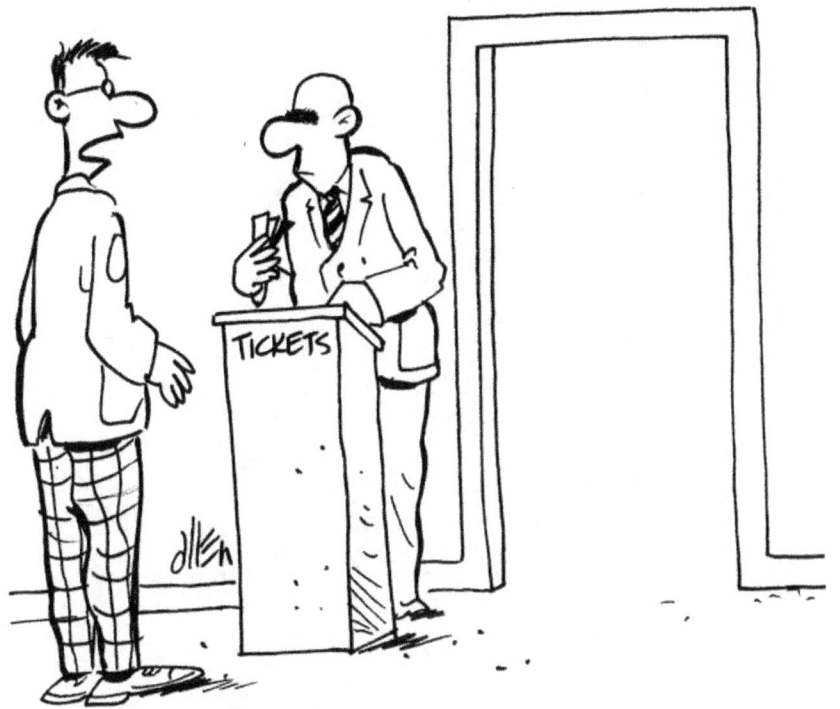

What!!.... you're charging us to attend the
monthly staff cost containment meeting.

Enter your caption:

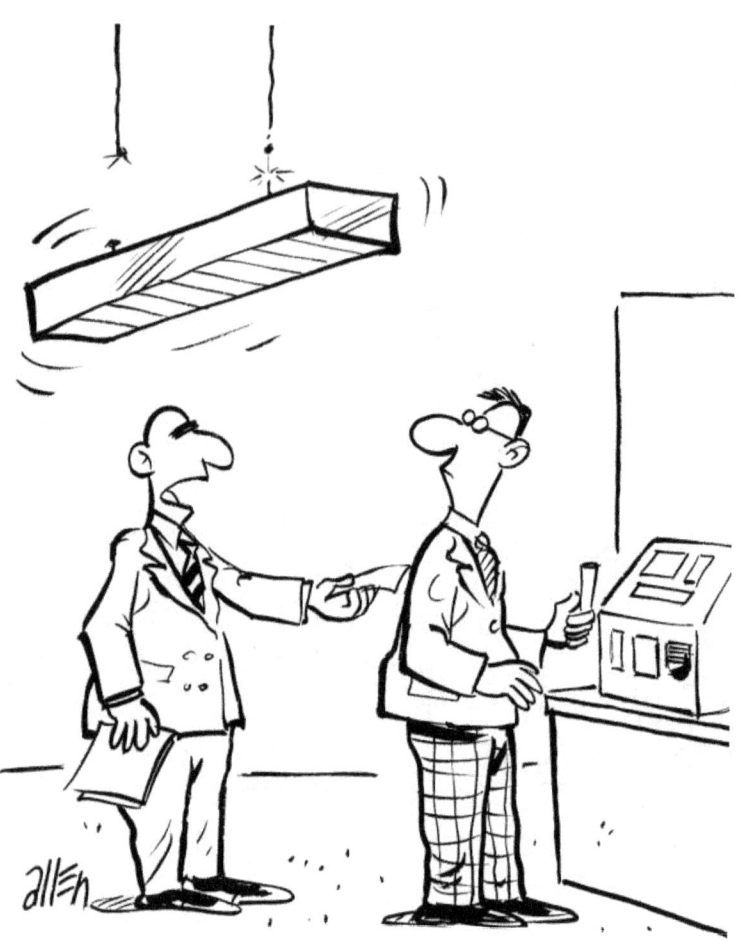

Here…I'm returning your repair request on the light. Incidental repairs are not a priority…unless they are life threatening.

Enter your caption:

_____

_____

_____

_____

_____

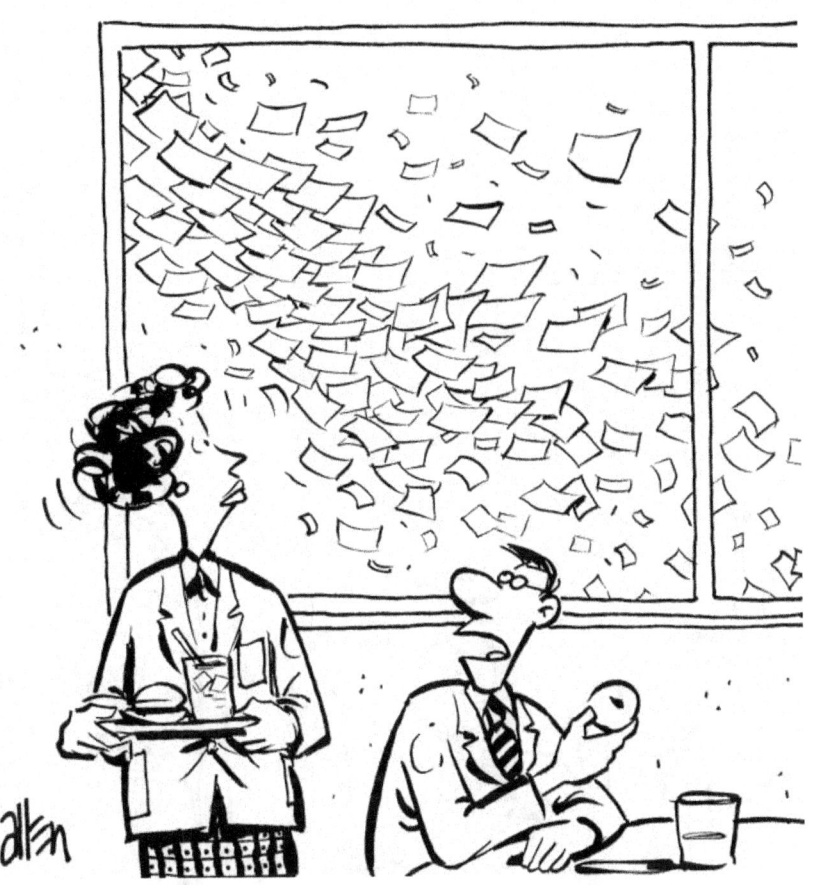

Ergo said to tell you he had a little accident with your fan...and wanted to know if the stack of papers next to it were very important.

Enter your caption:

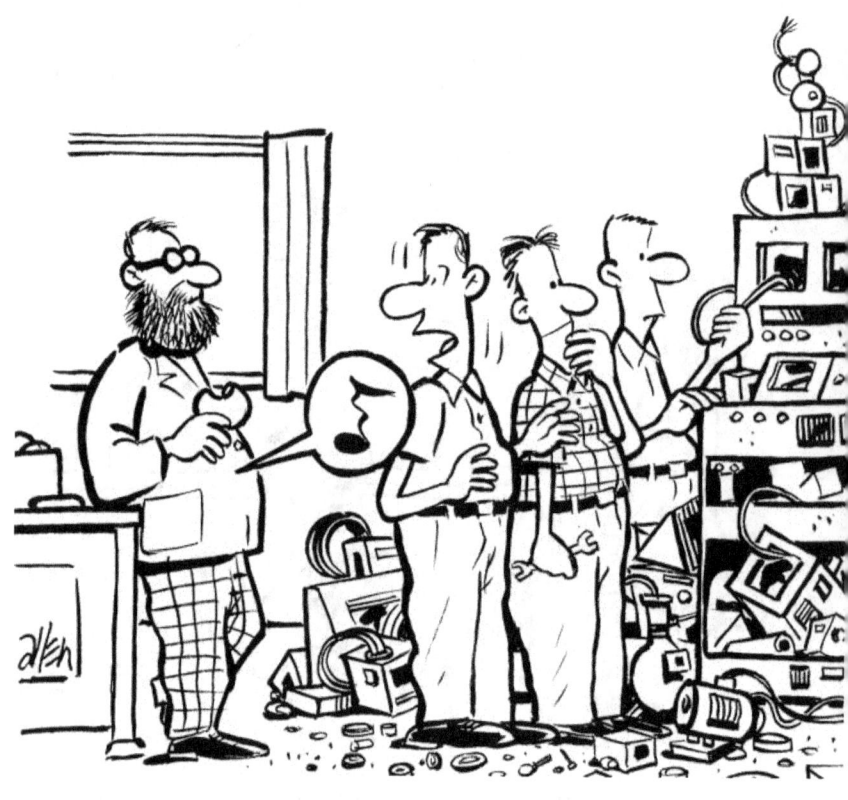

Wait a minute! That noise was NOT coming from
the monitor.

Enter your caption:

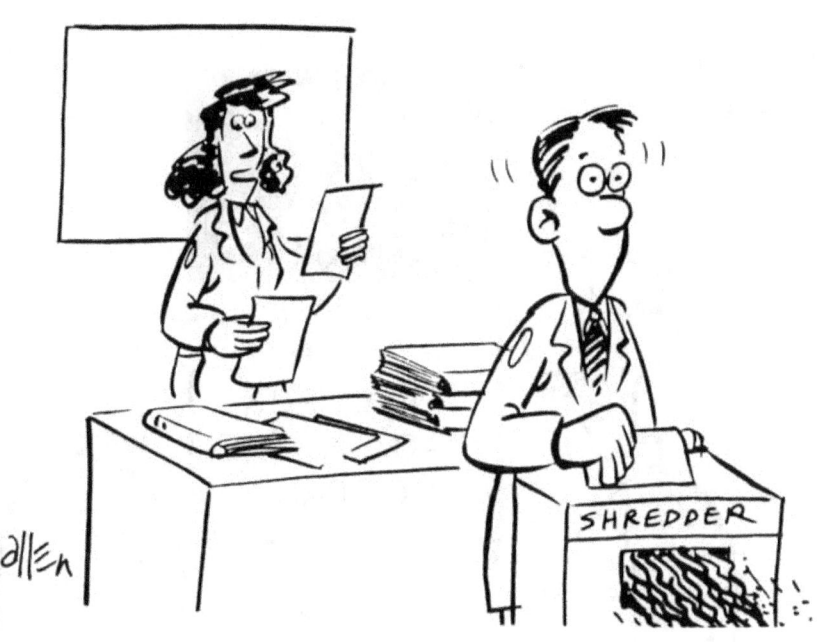

Uh oh…I mistakenly switched the "inbox" with the "to shred box."

Enter your caption:

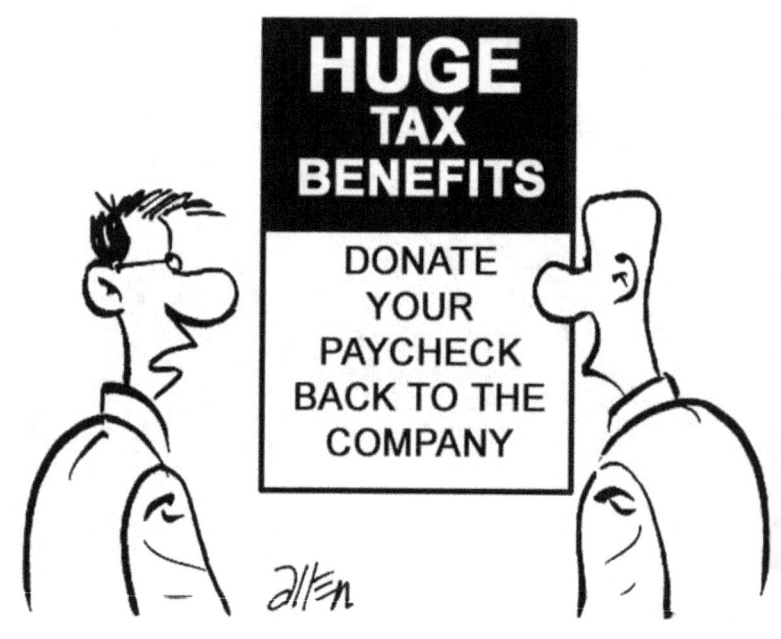

Business is bad…I suspect.

Enter your caption:

_____

_____

_____

_____

_____

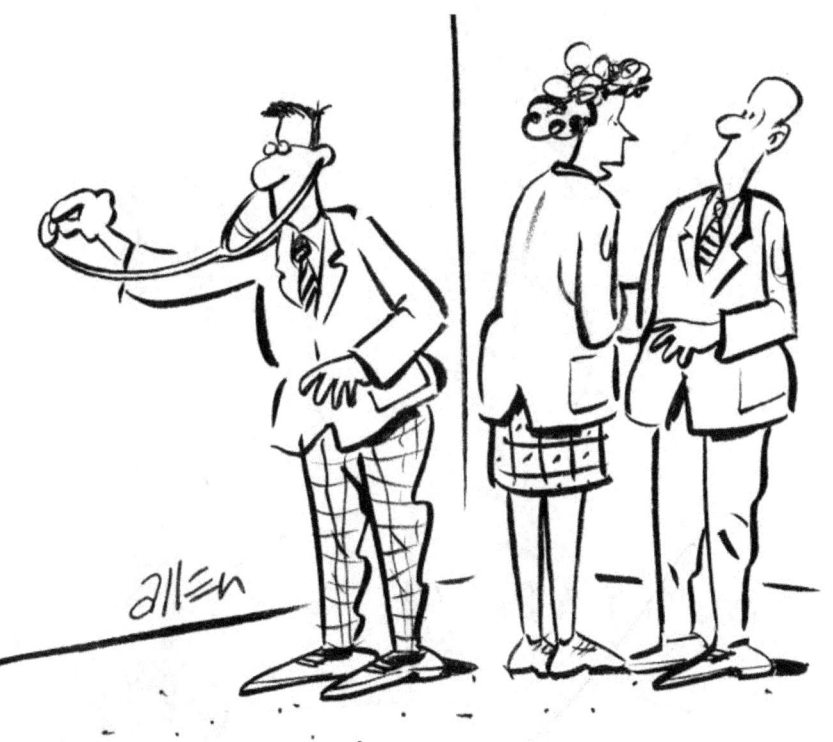

Must be another closed-door meeting!

Enter your caption:

_____

_____

_____

_____

_____

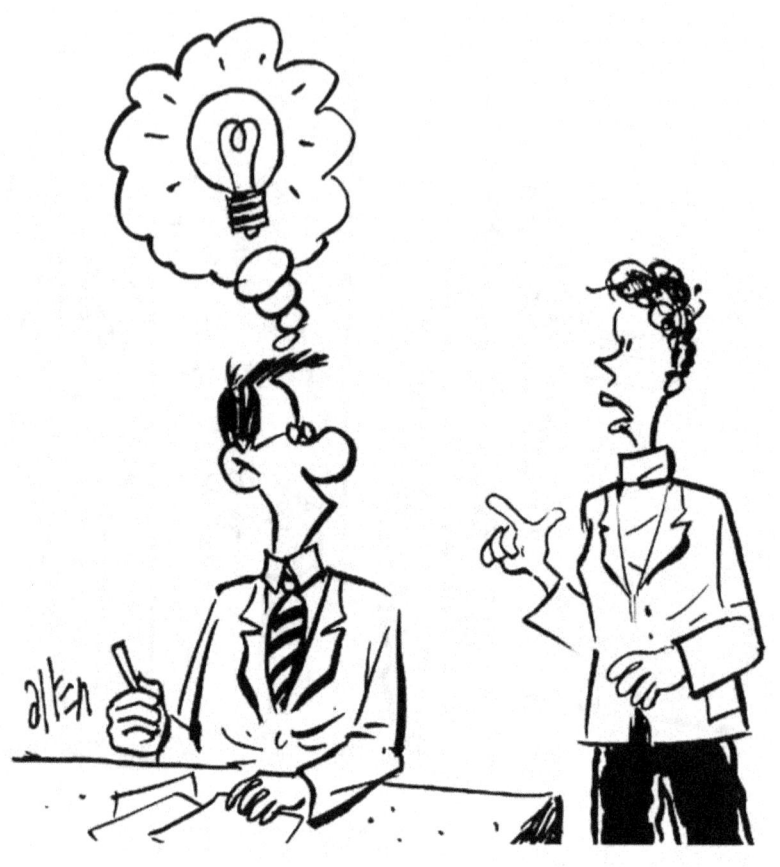

Look at you!! You're not using the new energy
efficient light bulb for your idea metaphor!!

Enter your caption:

_____

_____

_____

_____

_____

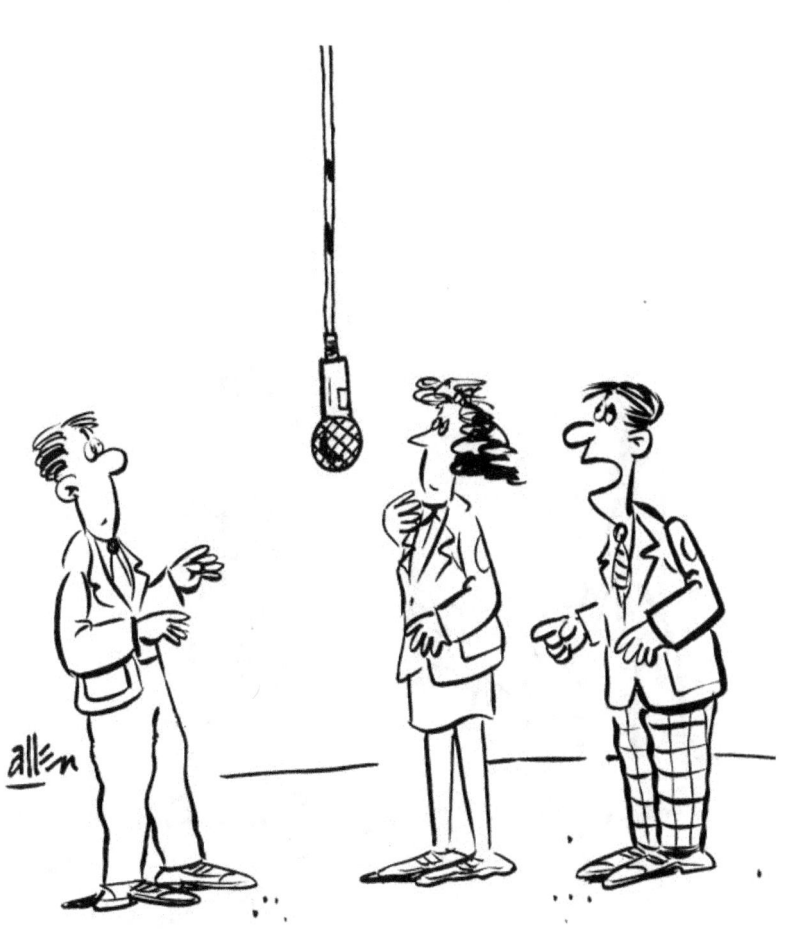

Just why do you think our boss is listening in
on our conversations.

Enter your caption:

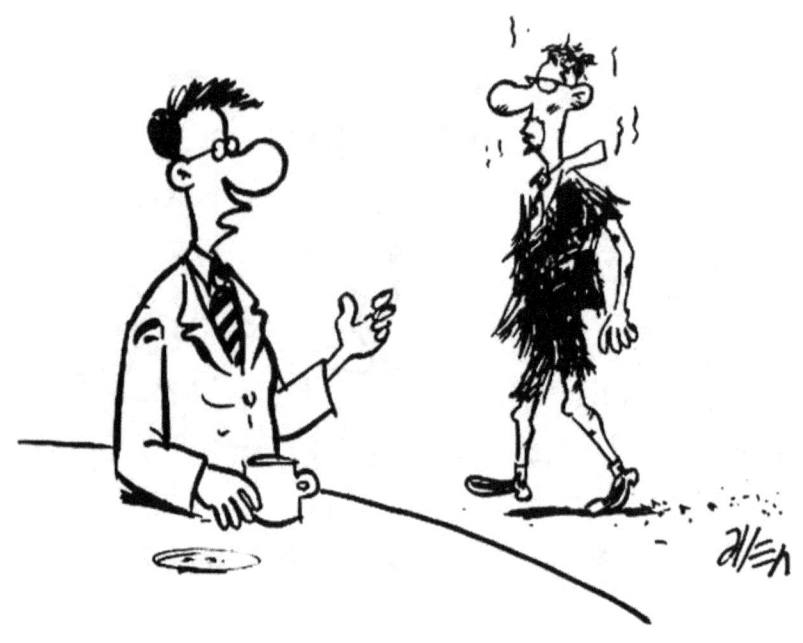

Oh…by the way, I think there might be a short in
one of our machines.

Enter your caption:

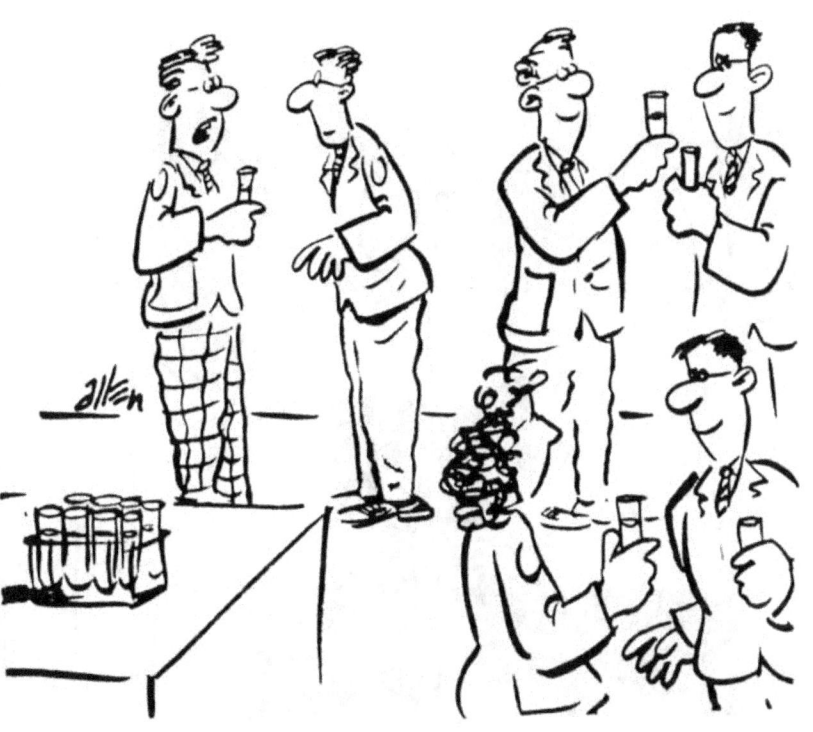

It's our weekly department party…Philpot
forgot the glasses!

Enter your caption:

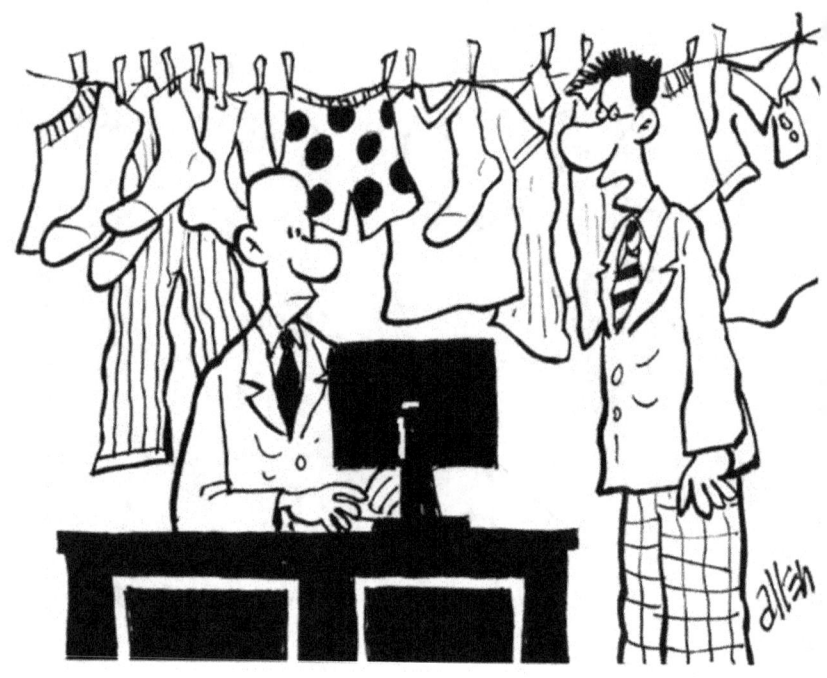

When was the last time you
clocked out?

Enter your caption:

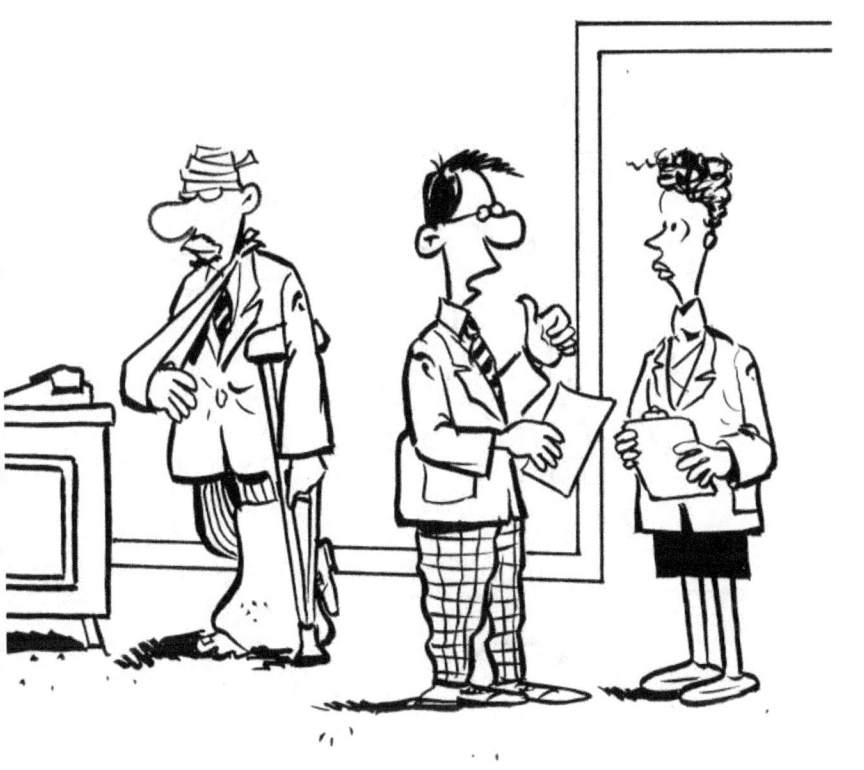

Ergo was reading a flow chart and the arrows
made him dizzy.

Enter your caption:

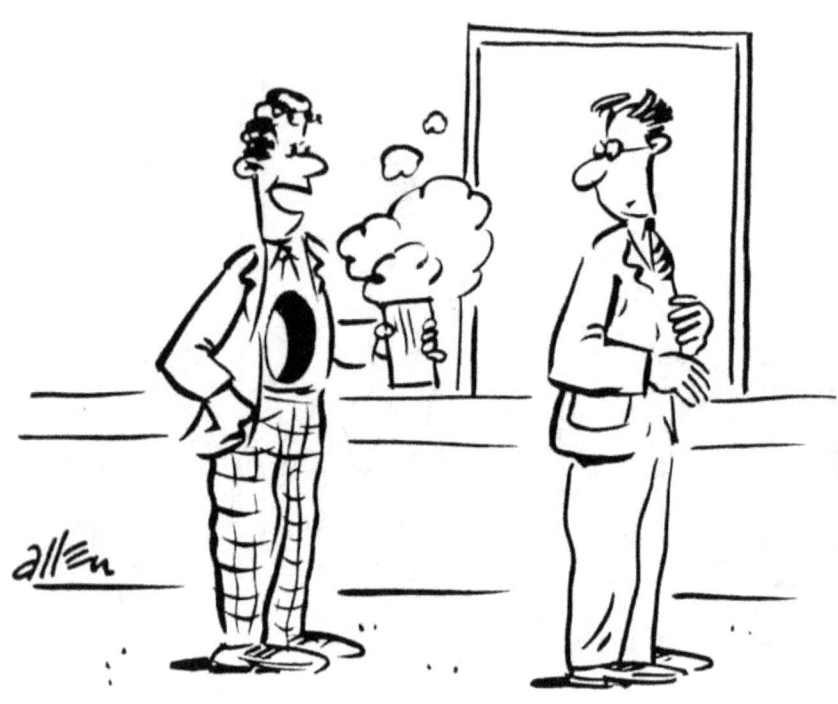

Hey Herb, I'll bet you can't guess who grabbed the liquid 02 instead of their pistachio malt.

Enter your caption:

_____

_____

_____

_____

_____

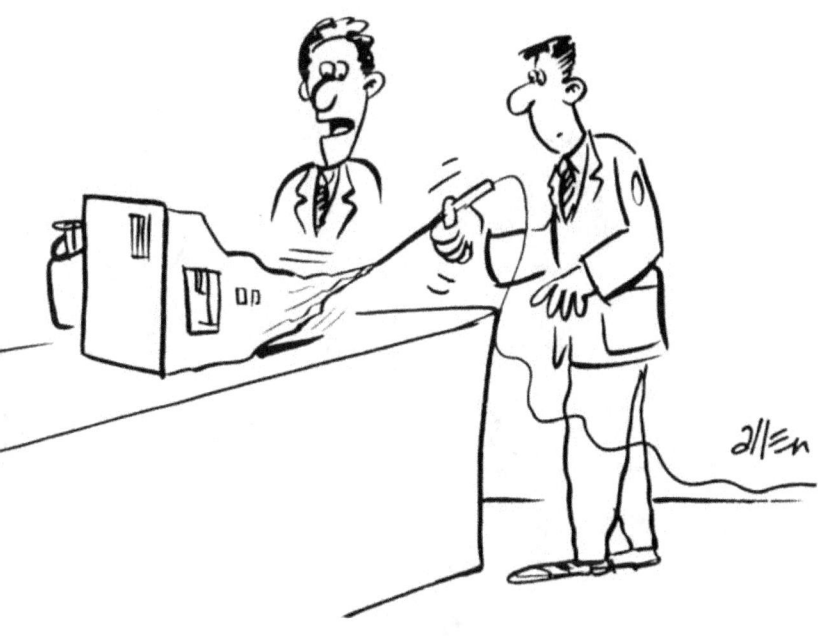

Whoa...pull back on the pipette...what negative
pressure did you use?

Enter your caption:

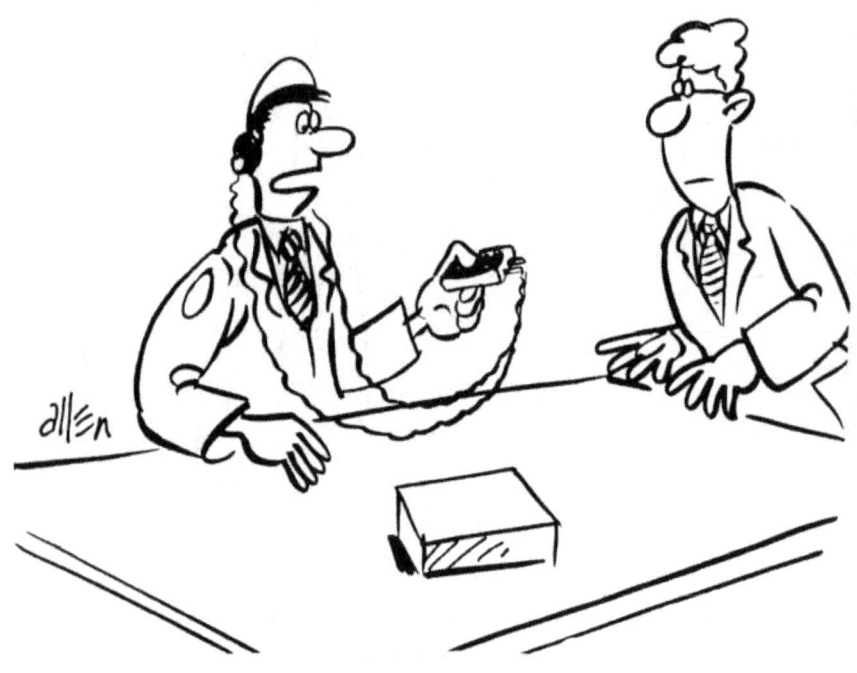

I hate it when Gardenia gives the report with
sound effects.

Enter your caption:

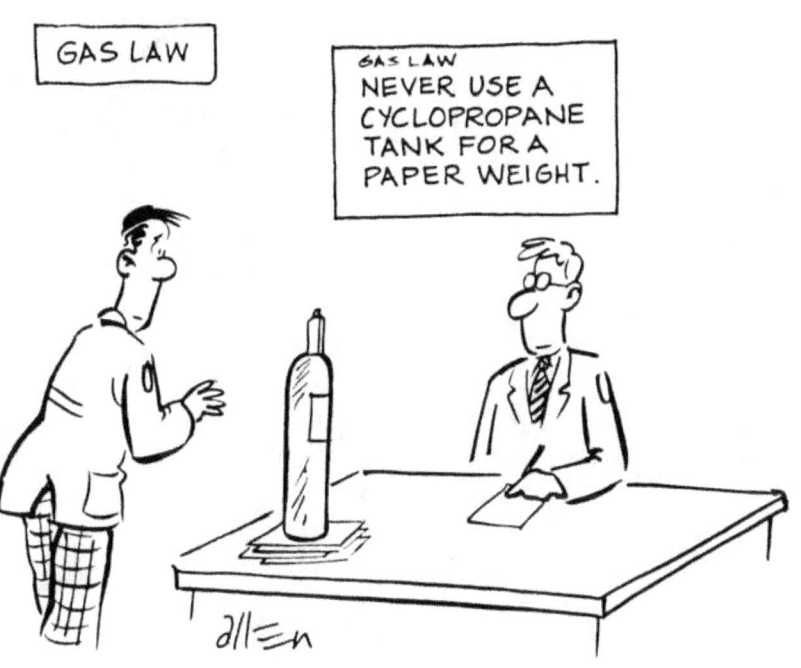

Stewart lived on the edge.

Enter your caption:

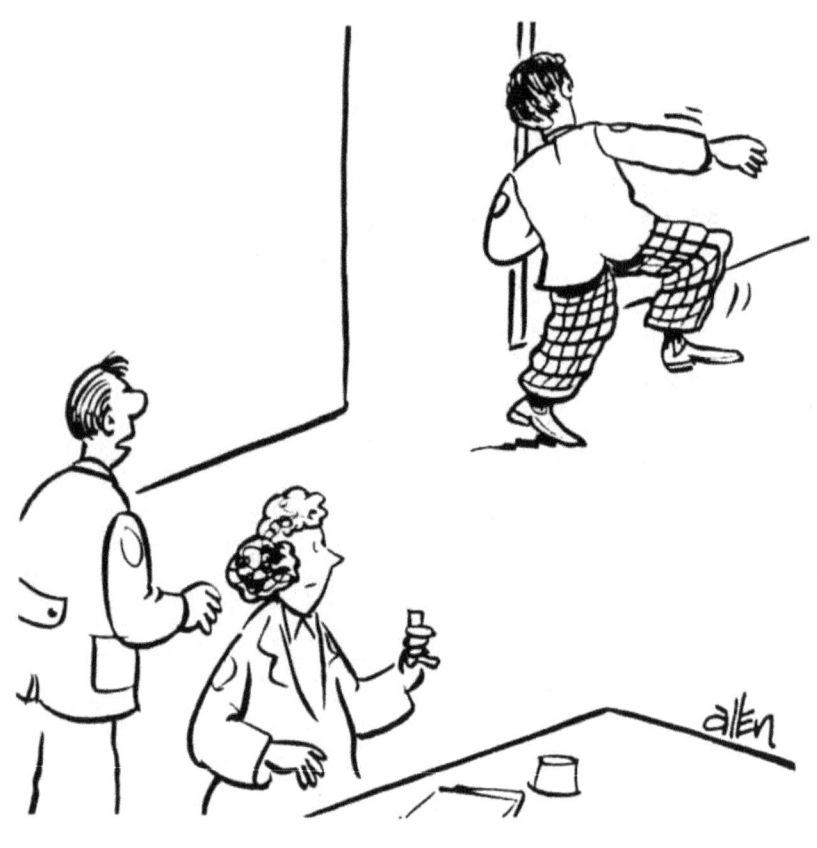

Ozzie must have been staring at the
centrifuge again.

Enter your caption:

_____

_____

_____

_____

_____

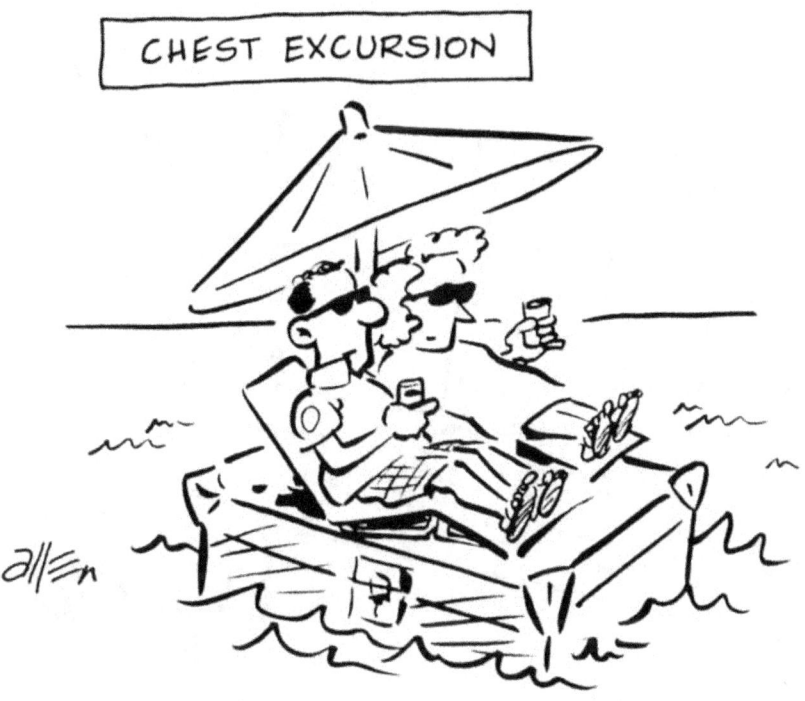

Pulmonologists Dr. Nod and Rocha's love of puns lead them to far away places.

Enter your caption:

_____

_____

_____

_____

_____

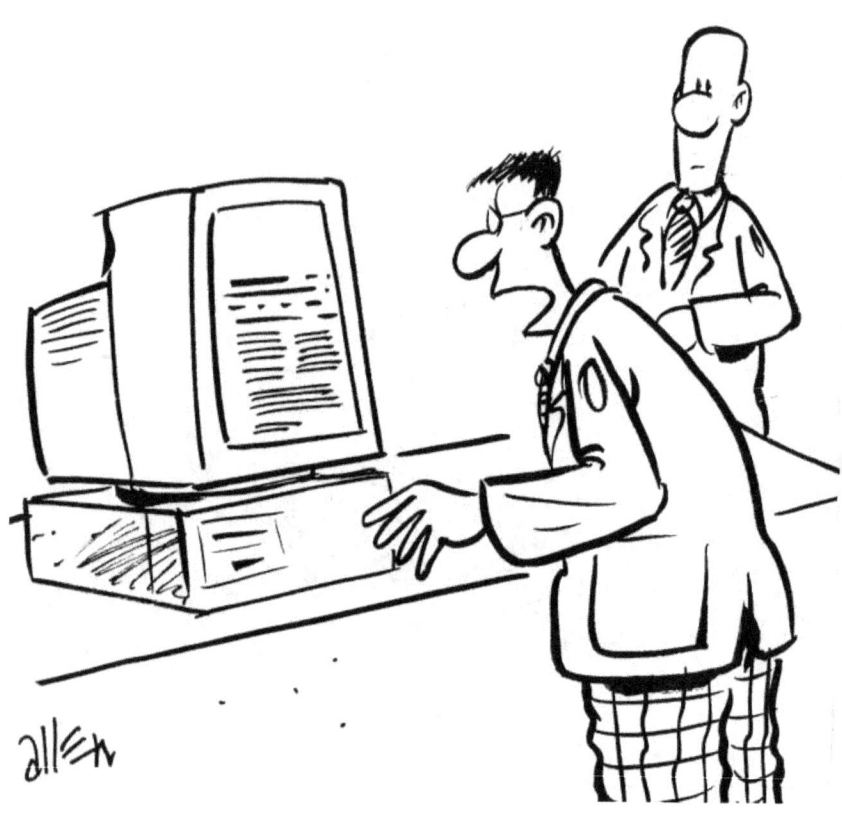

I'm trying to retrieve some data, but I keep getting the false promises of elected officials.

Enter your caption:

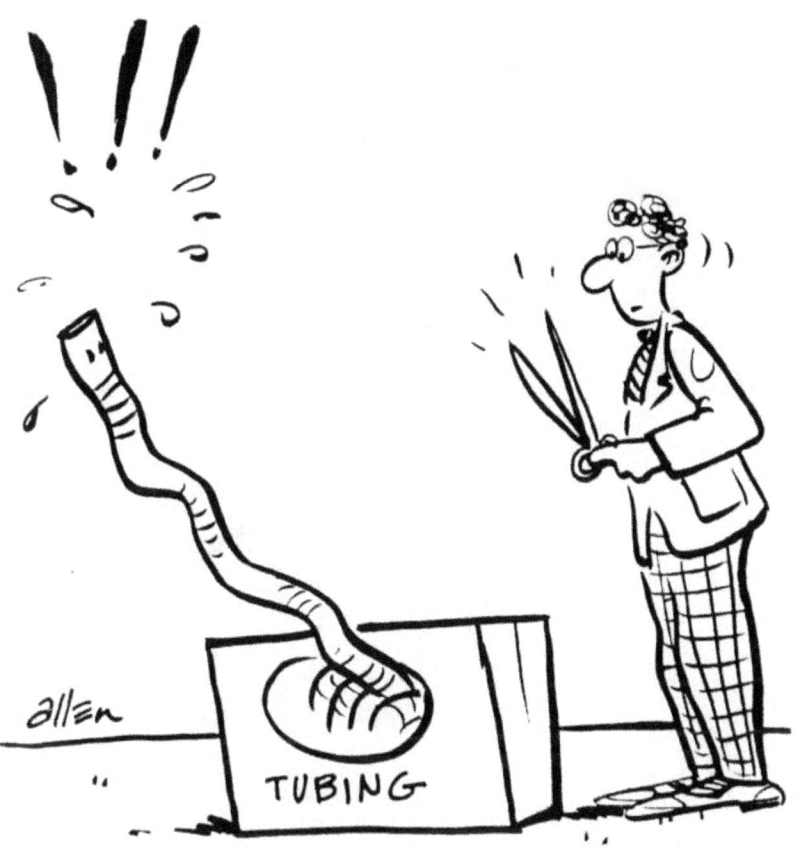

Cutting tubing was a part of Mark's everyday routine in Respiratory Therapy, but one day he saw life from a tube's perspective.

Enter your caption:

_____

_____

_____

_____

_____

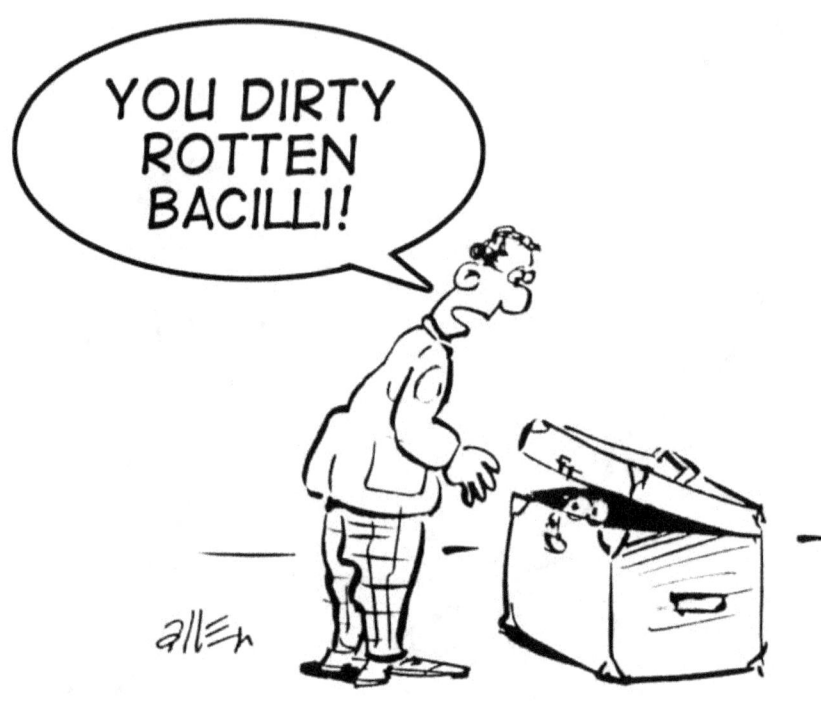

Dr. Crawford often gave a metaphorical portrayal
of a love-hate relationship between a doctor
and a germ.

Enter your caption:

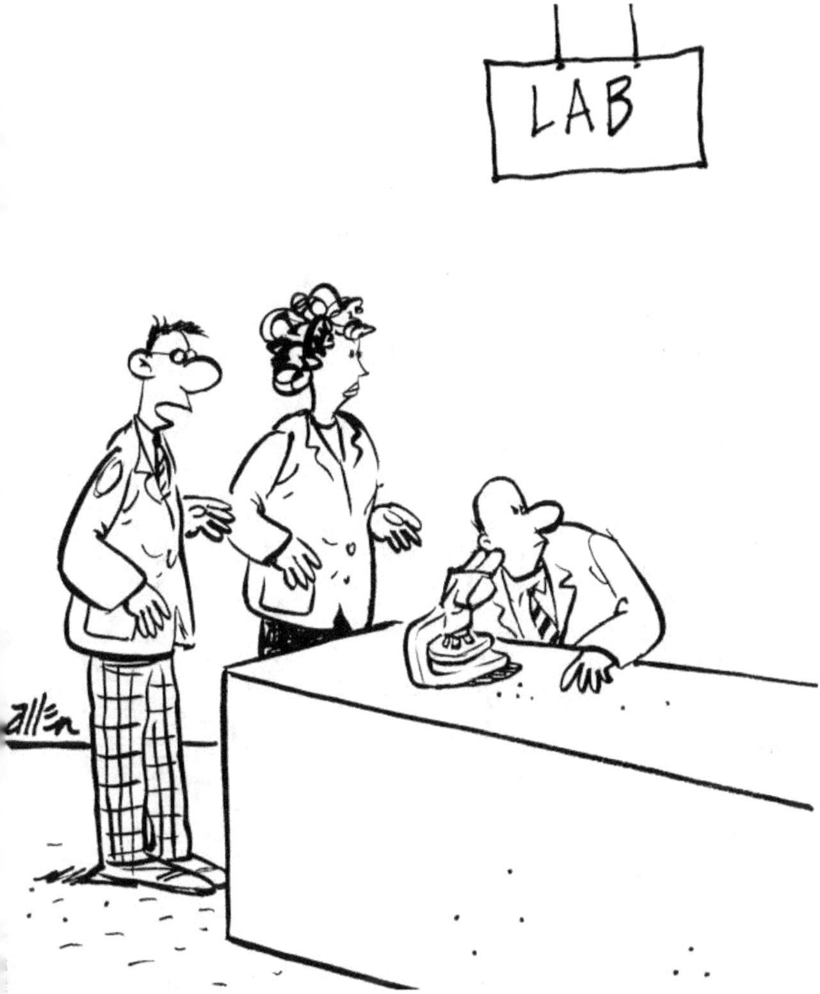

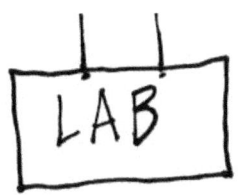

He swears up and down that it said something to him.

Enter your caption:

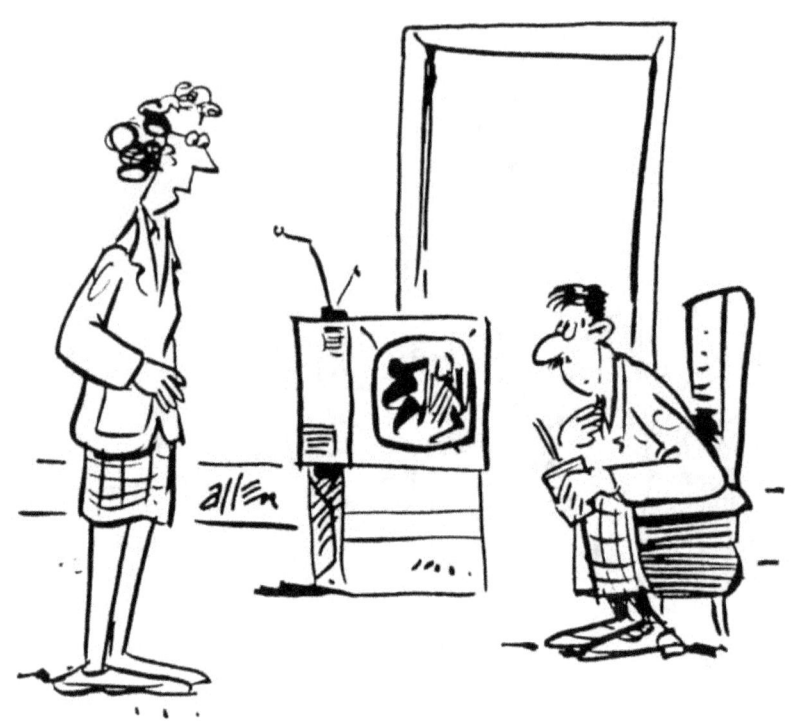

No...I don't think watching Scrubs
re-runs will count towards CEUs.

Enter your caption:

_____

_____

_____

_____

_____

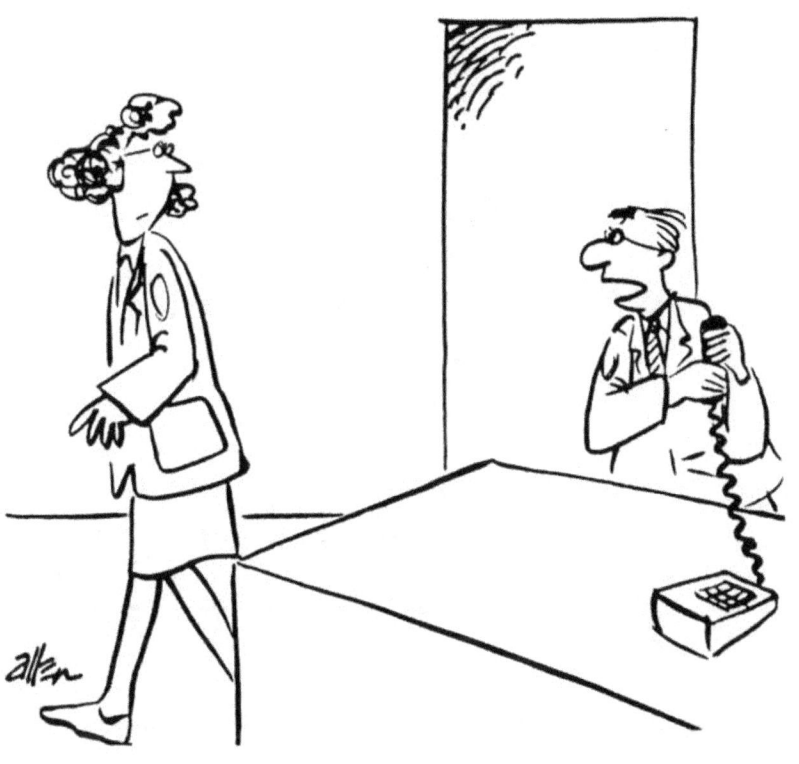

Four-south wants to know what we can do for a
nose out of joint.

Enter your caption:

_____

_____

_____

_____

_____

KREBS CYCLE

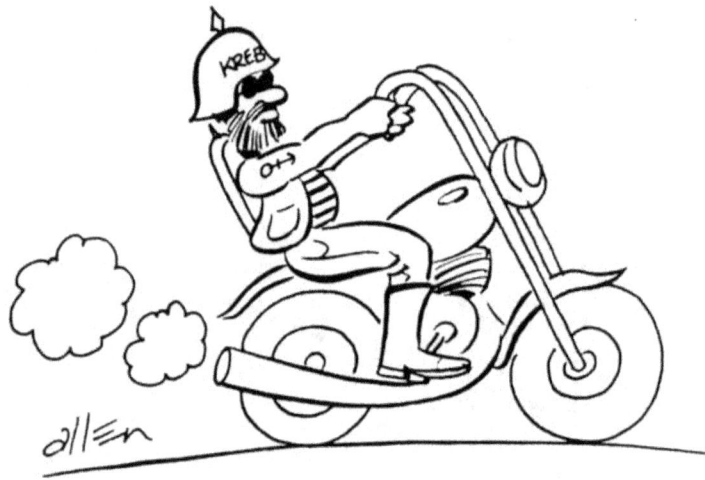

Hans Krebs, after his famous discovery about metabolic pathways in cells, couldn't take the grind in the animal lab so he dropped out with his hog.

Enter your caption:

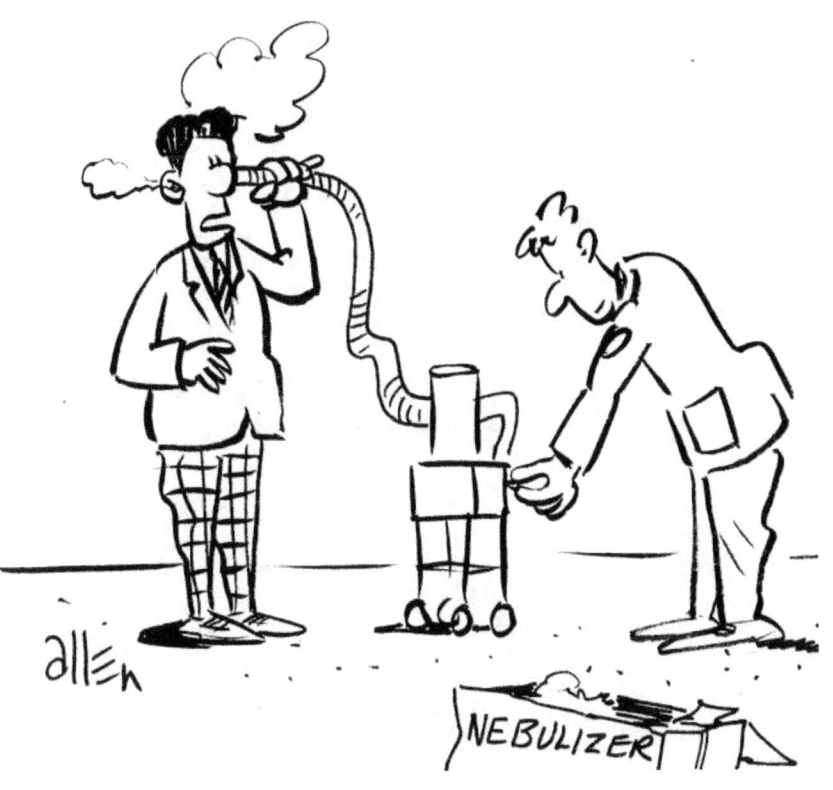

You're right...it does sound
like the ocean!

Enter your caption:

_____

_____

_____

_____

_____

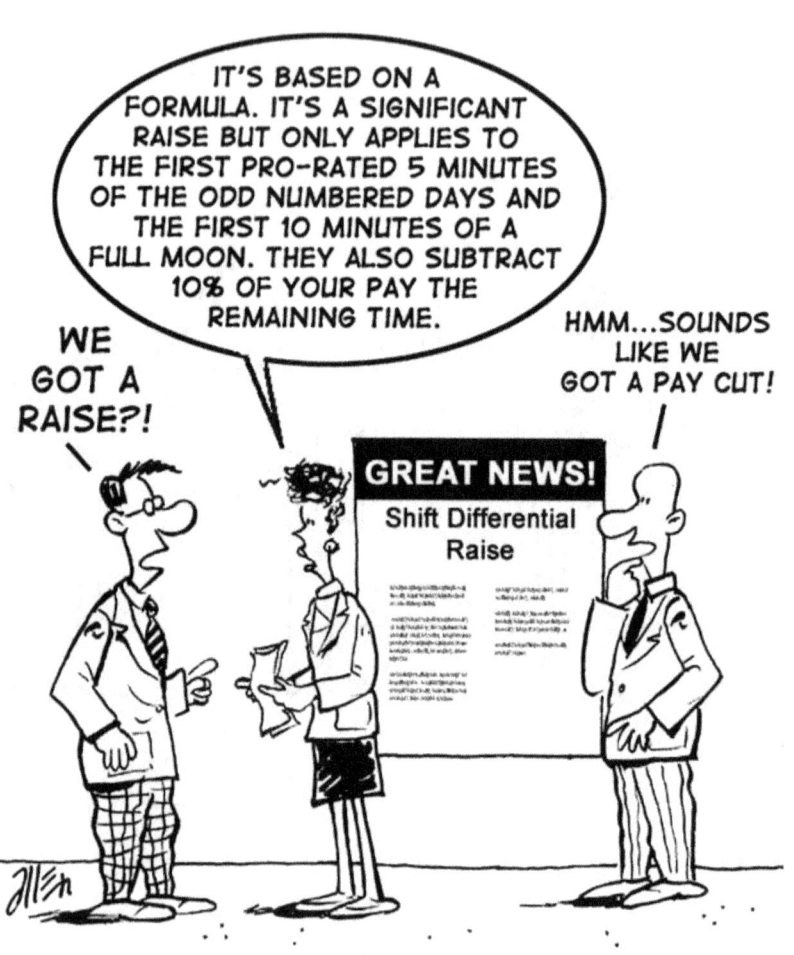

Enter your caption:

_____

_____

_____

_____

_____

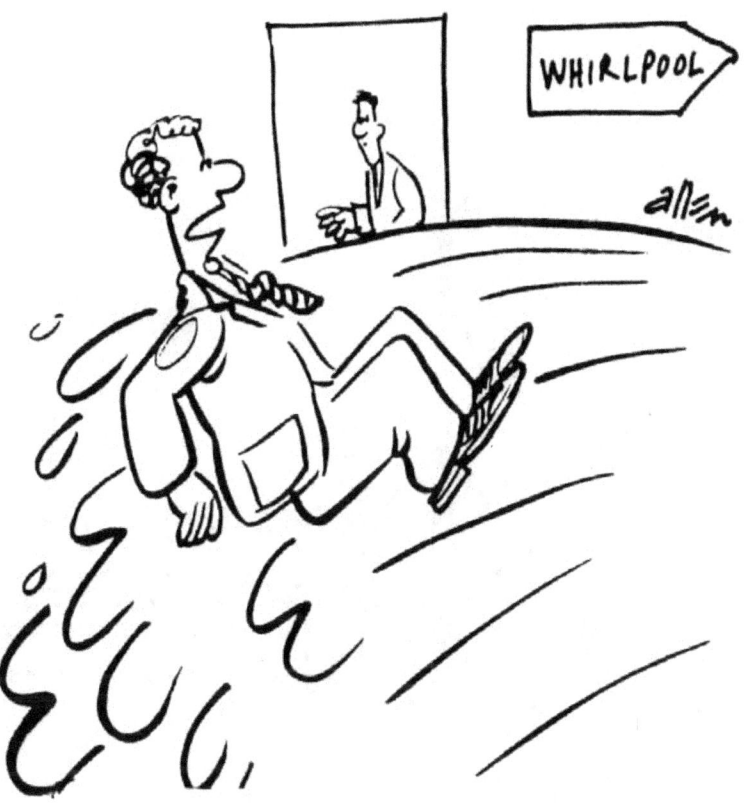

Oh…not bad, how's it going with you.

Enter your caption:

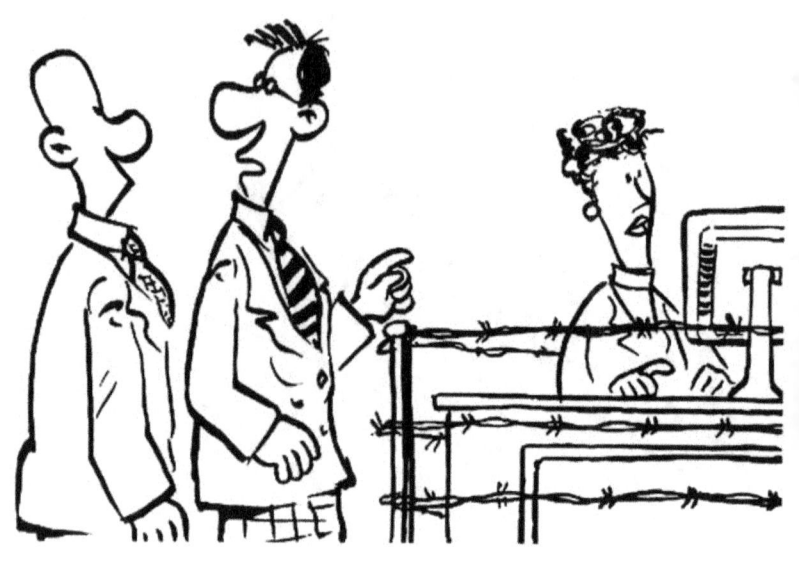

I think it means she doesn't want
to be bothered.

Enter your caption:

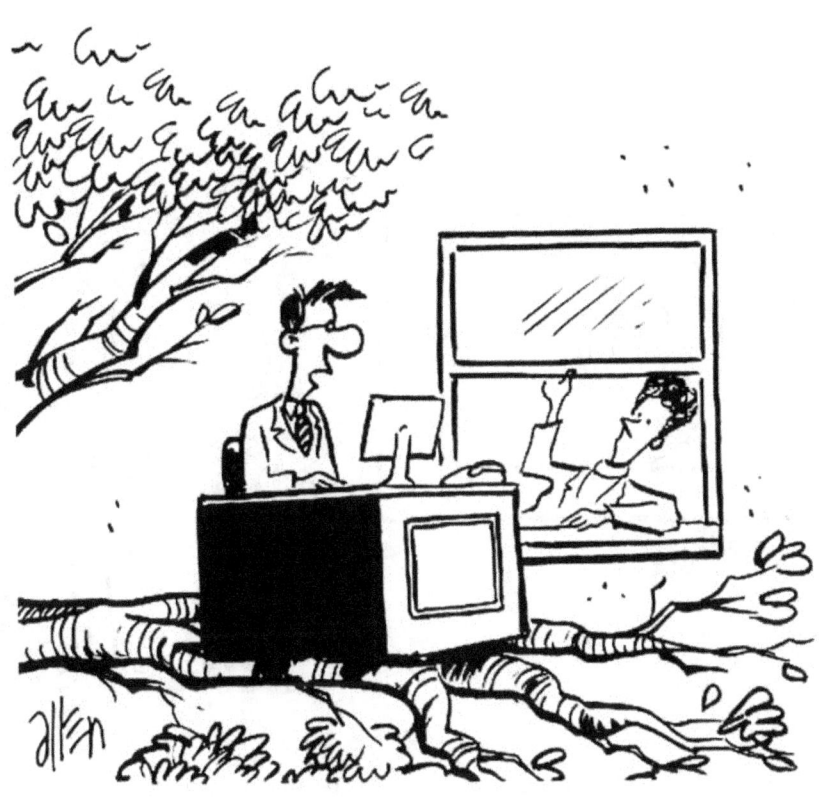

...and what makes you think I'm not a
TEAM PLAYER?

Enter your caption:

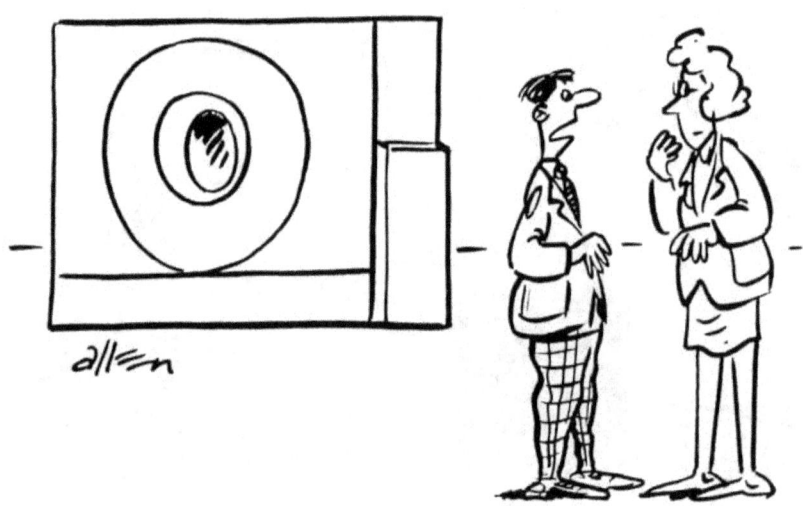

I know it looks like the CAT scan we ordered, but we found out it's a commercial washing machine.

Enter your caption:

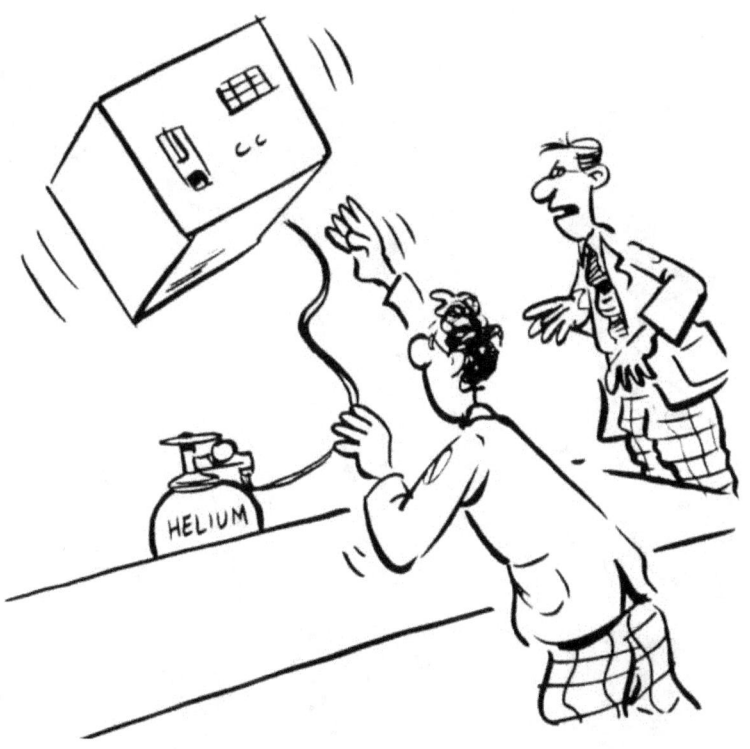

Did you hook up the wrong
test gas?

Enter your caption:

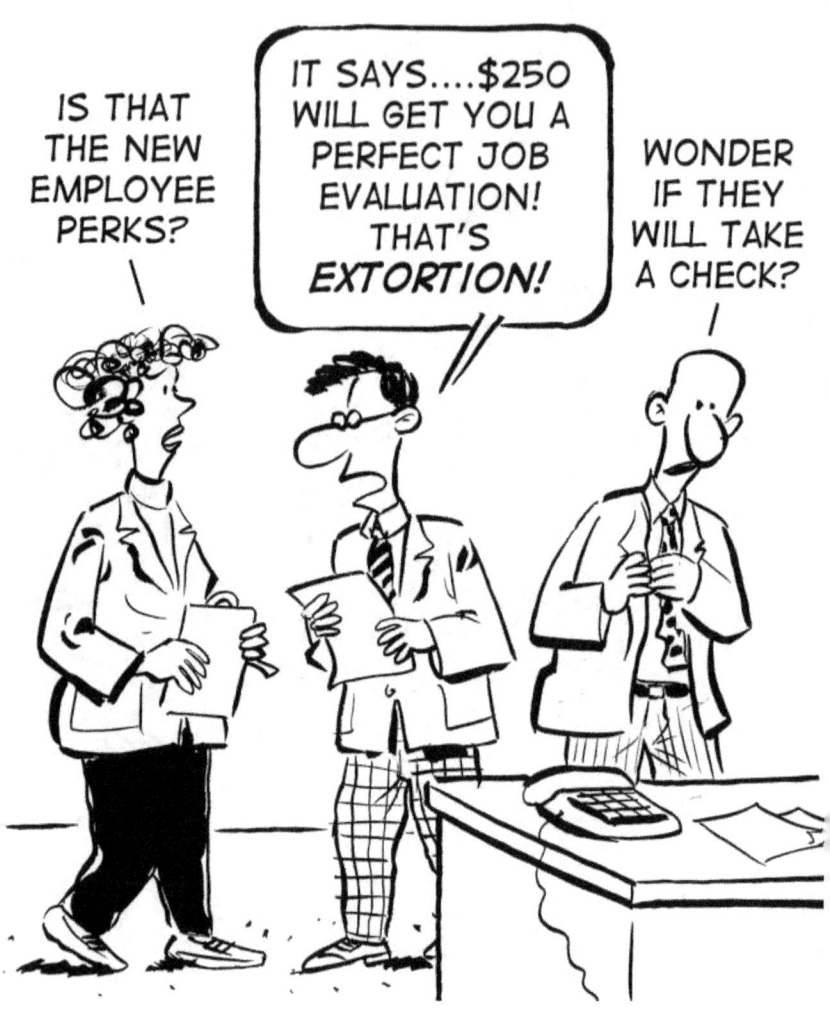

Enter your caption:

_____

_____

_____

_____

_____

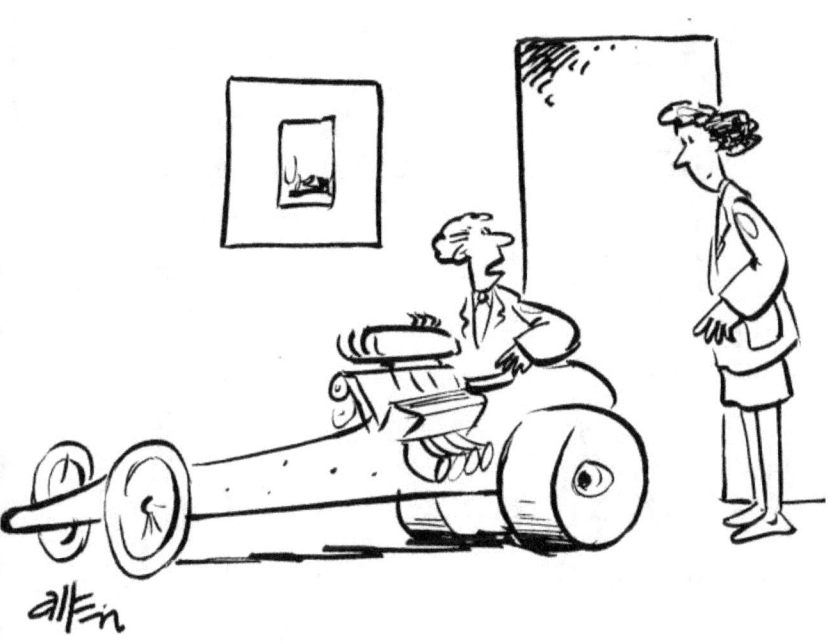

...it's for extra **extra** stat calls.

Enter your caption:

_____

_____

_____

_____

_____

_____

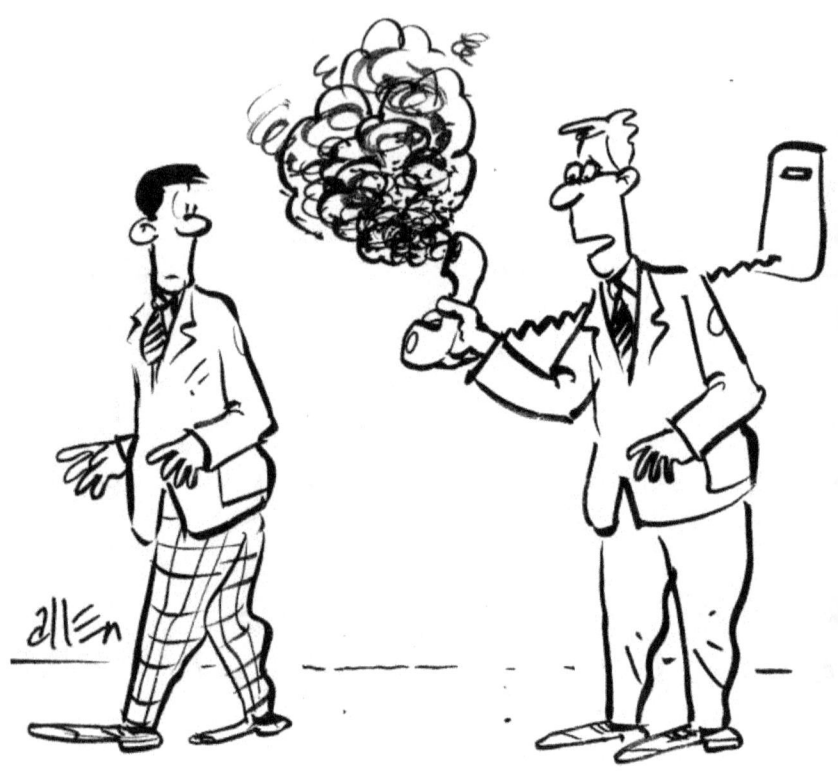

It's Mr. Smoka from the stop-smoking workshop and just wanted to update you on his progress.

Enter your caption:

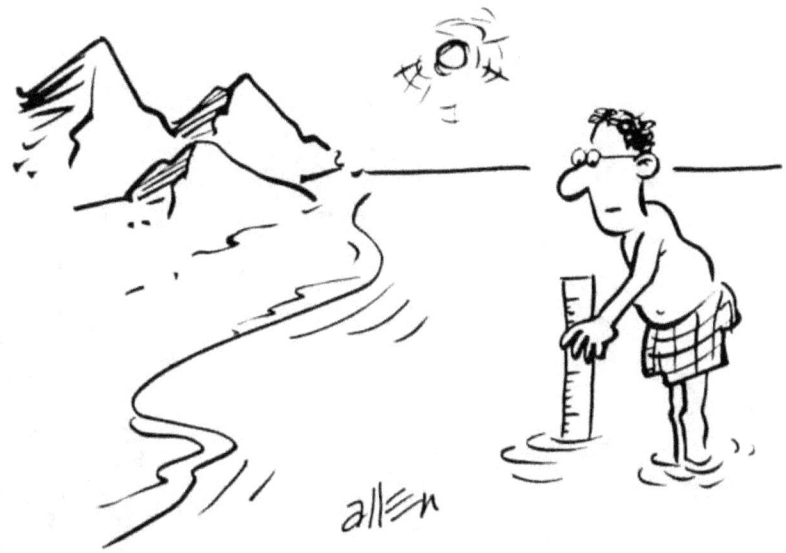

MEASURING TIDAL VOLUMES

Tony, when told to measure the tidal volumes on his floor, misunderstood and went to Belize.

Enter your caption:

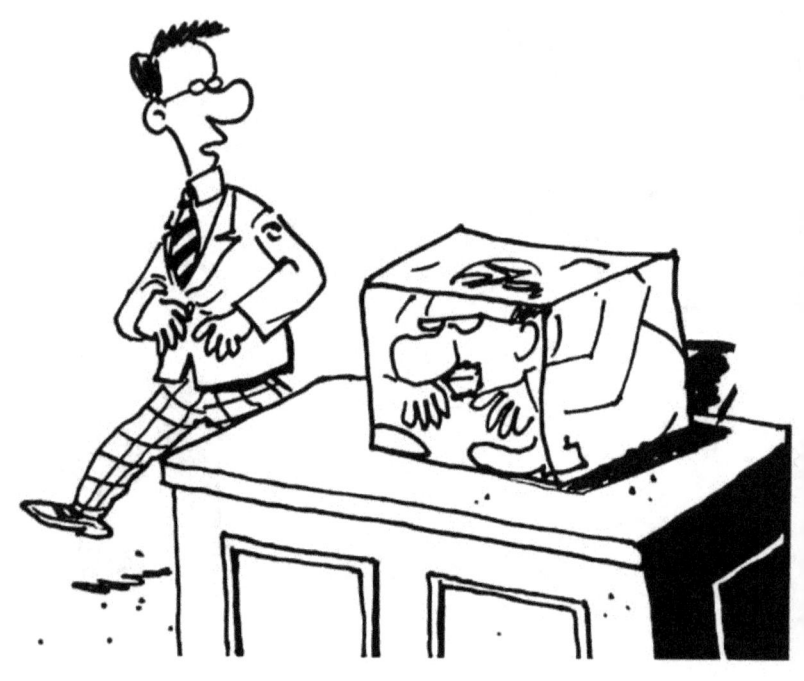

Oh, hi Ergo…I see you've fixed the trash
compactor.

Enter your caption:

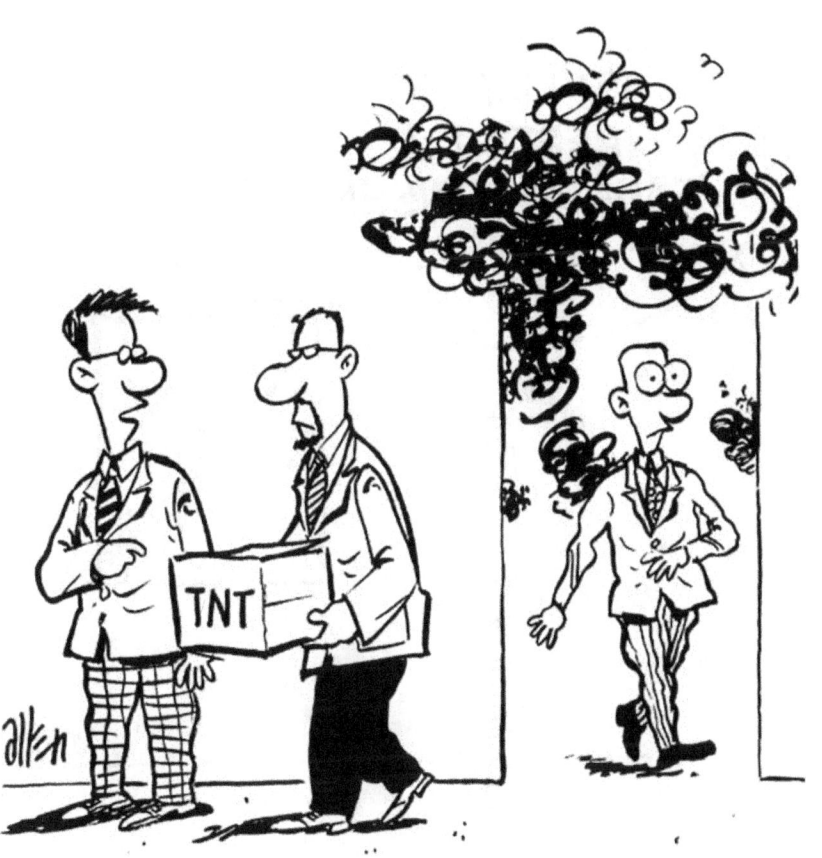

Not one person slept through your
Power Point!

Enter your caption:

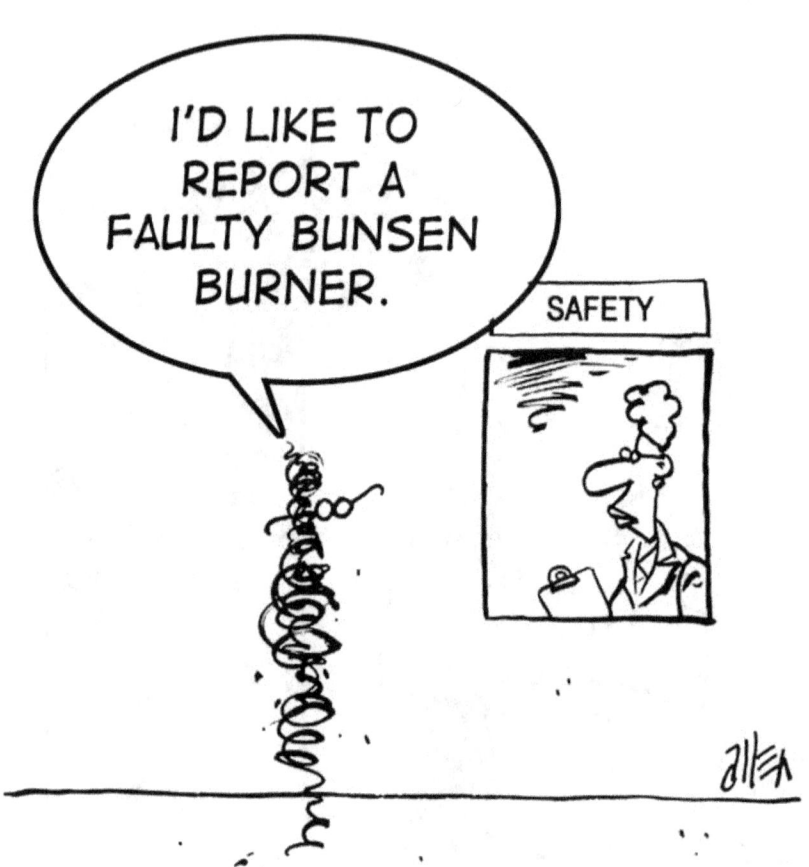

Enter your caption:

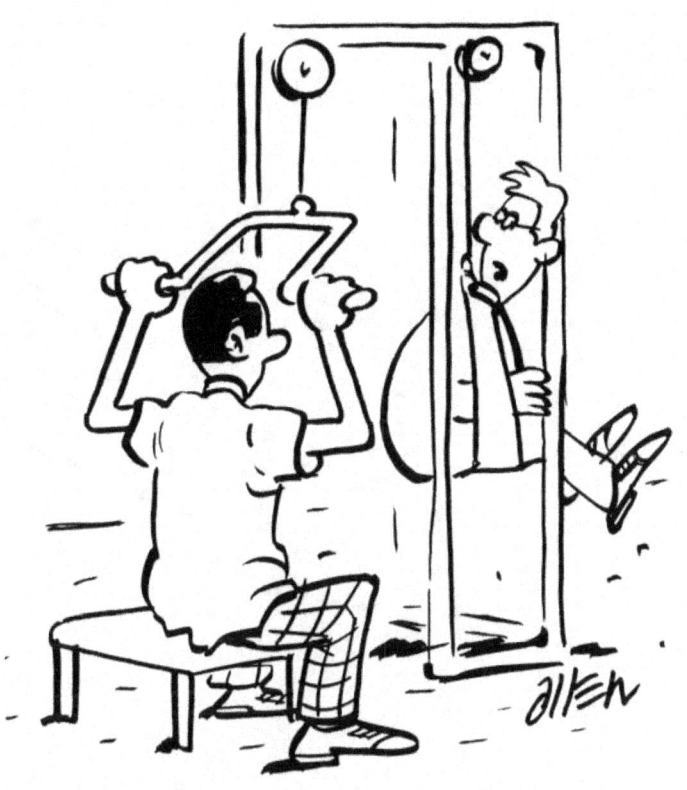

The weights have not come in yet...
so I'm filling in.

Enter your caption:

LARGE BORE TUBE

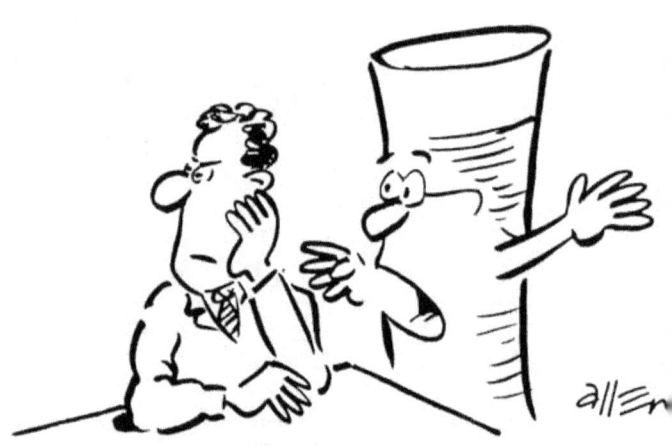

After hearing one too many talking tubes, Art
realized he had been working too many hours
and needed some time off.

Enter your caption:

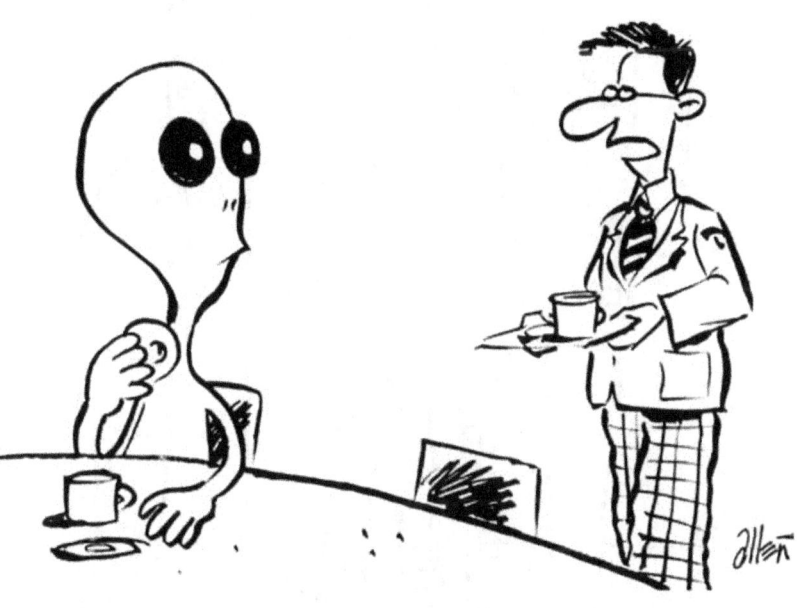

You must be the new employee
everyone is talking about.

Enter your caption:

_____

_____

_____

_____

_____

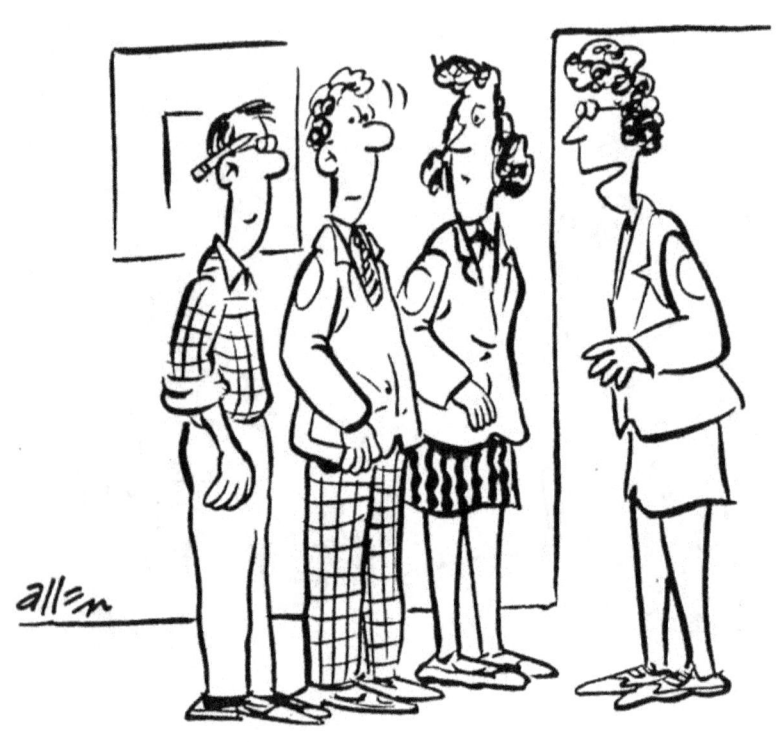

Our x-ray unit is down, but do not fear…a
cartoonist is here.

Enter your caption:

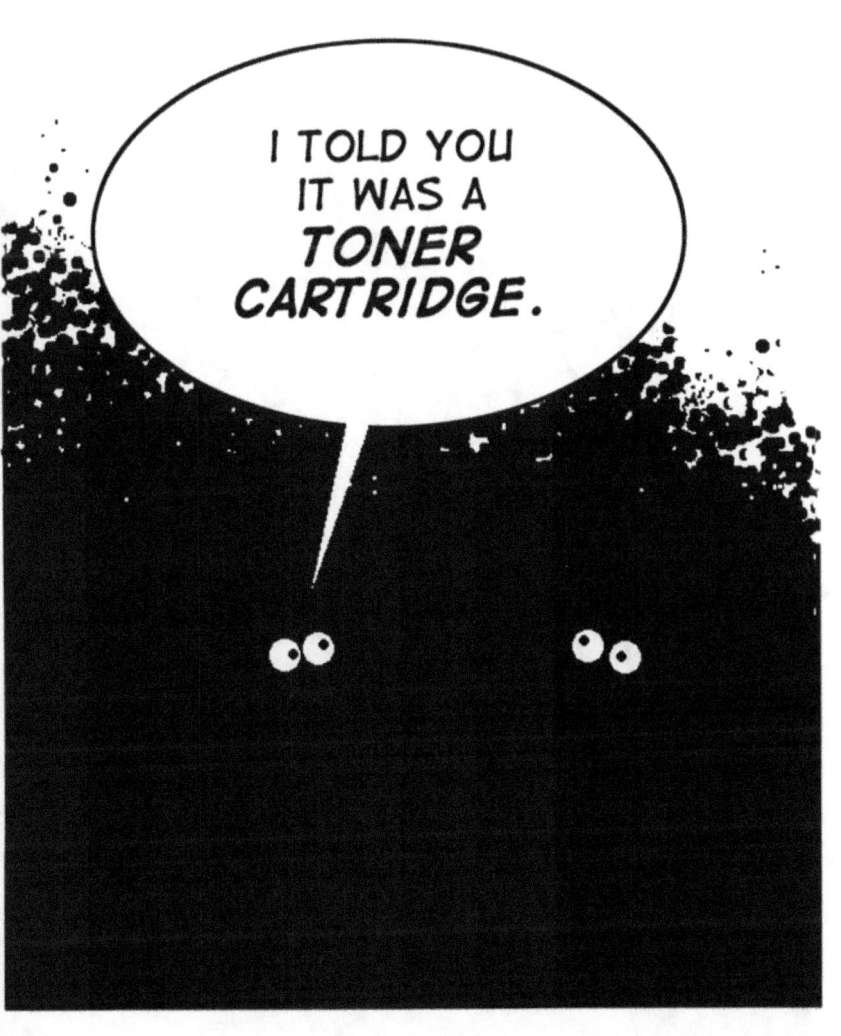

Enter your caption:

_____

_____

_____

_____

_____

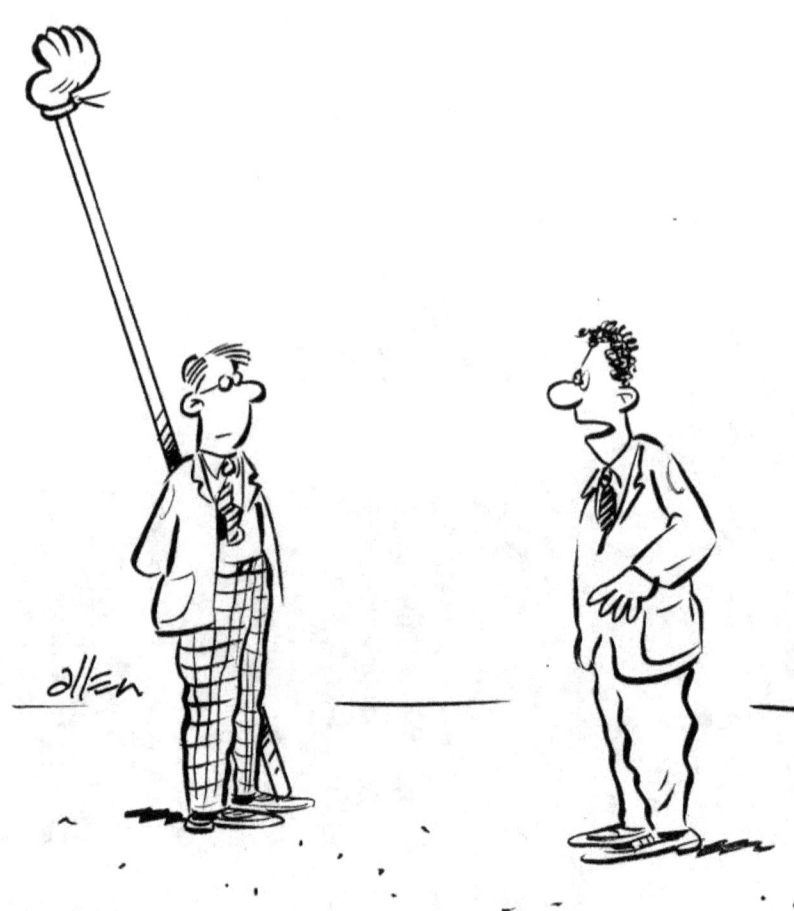

I'm sorry, but that won't work! You have to
actually go into the isolation room.

Enter your caption:

_____

_____

_____

_____

_____

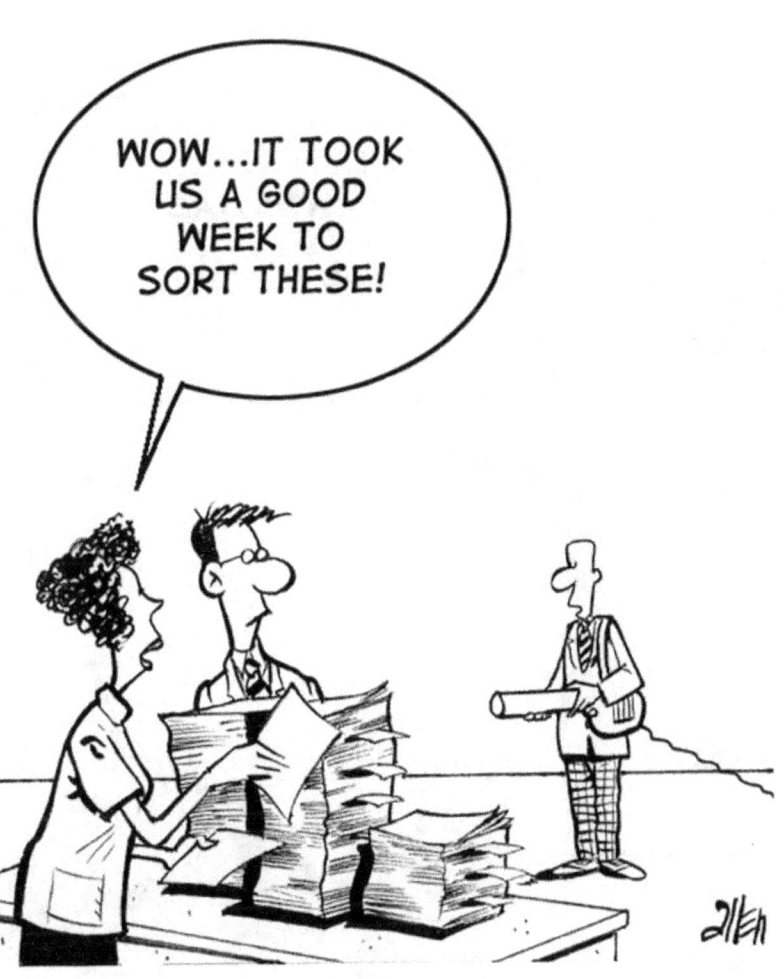

Hey guys, check out the velocity
on this.

Enter your caption:

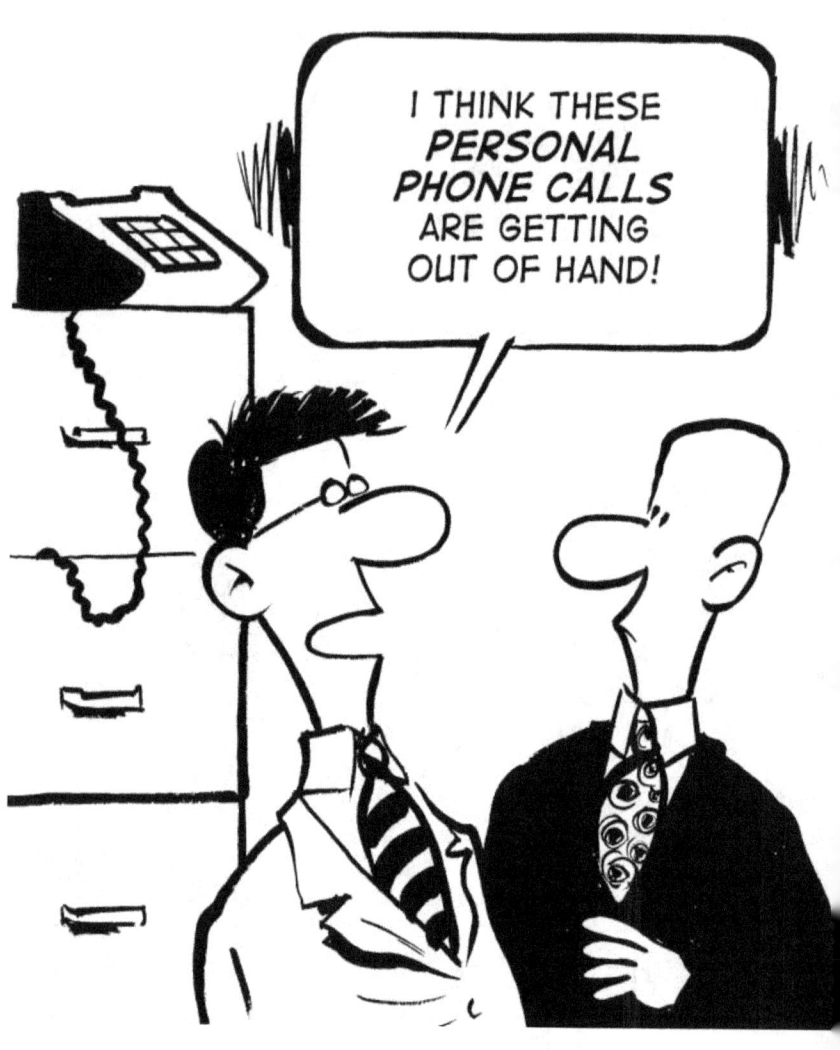

Enter your caption:

_____

_____

_____

_____

_____

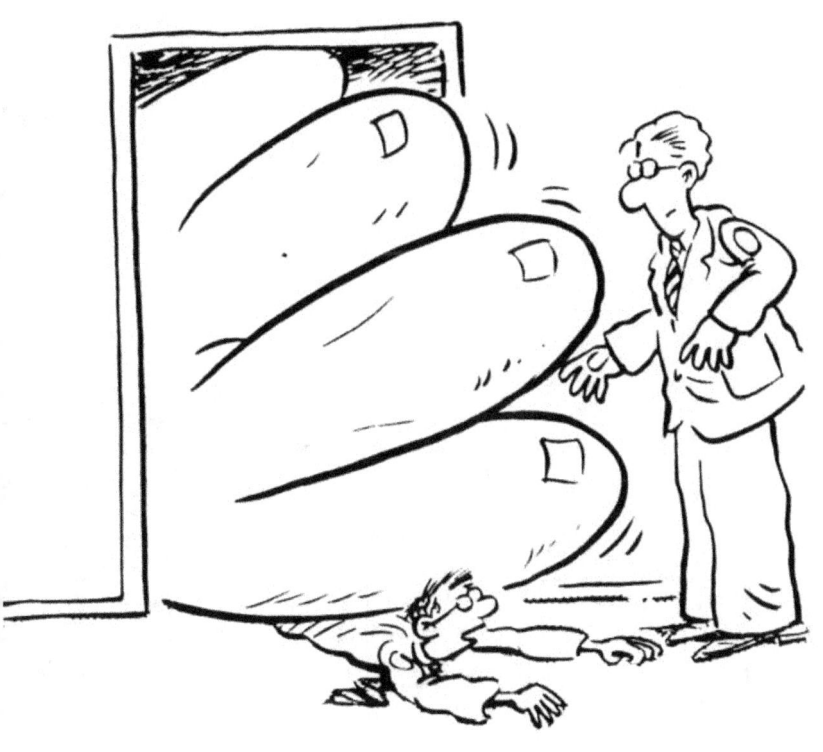

I just wanted to see how big I could get this exam
glove on the helium tank.

Enter your caption:

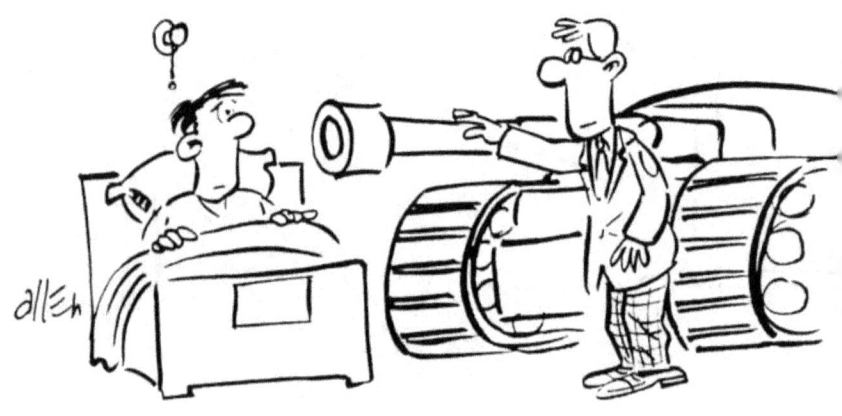

Lars, on his first day on the job, messed up big time.

Enter your caption:

_____

_____

_____

_____

_____

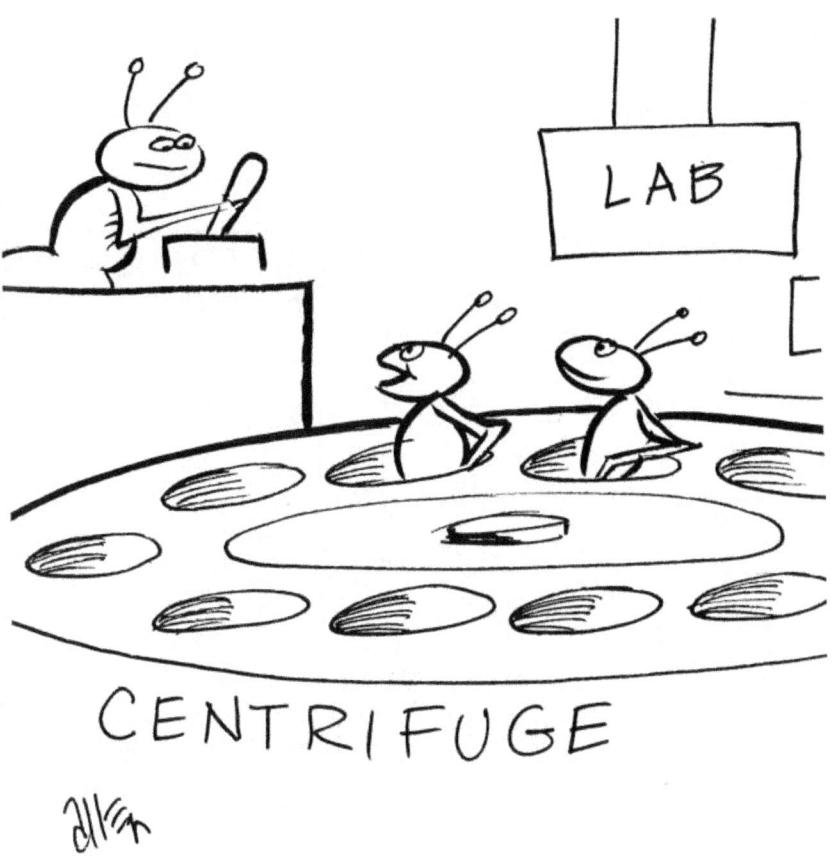

OK....turn it on!!

Enter your caption:

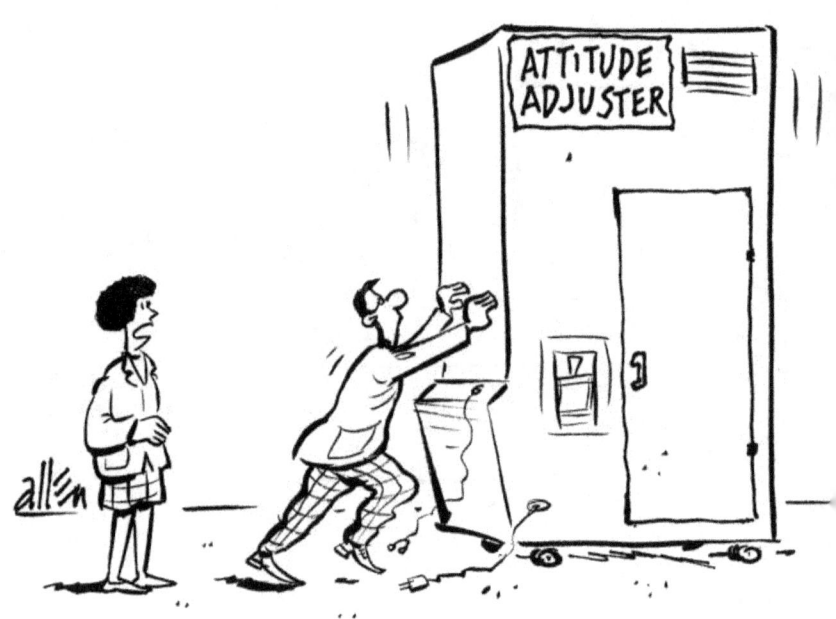

I'll bet you got some big time morale
problems in your department!

Enter your caption:

_____

_____

_____

_____

_____

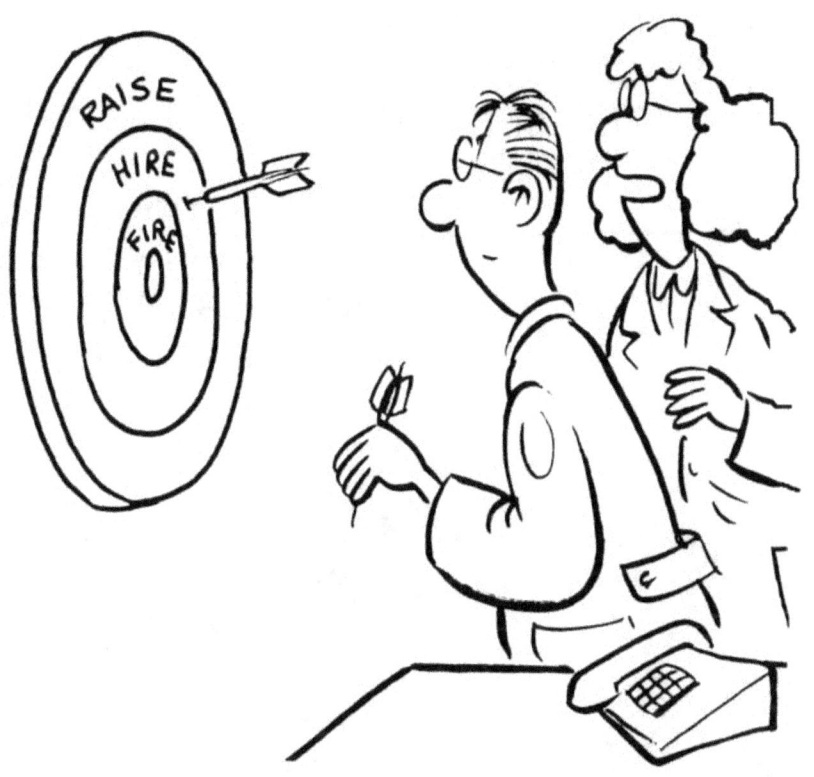

Wow...I thought there was more to
management than this.

Enter your caption:

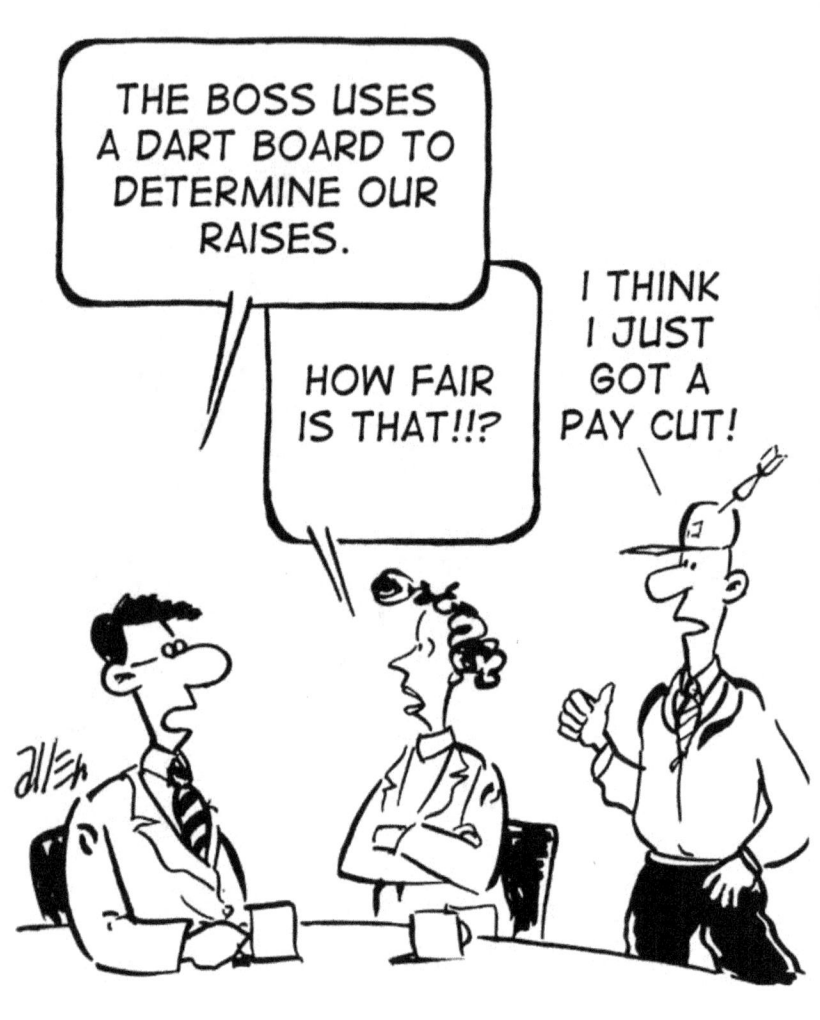

Enter your caption:

_____

_____

_____

_____

_____

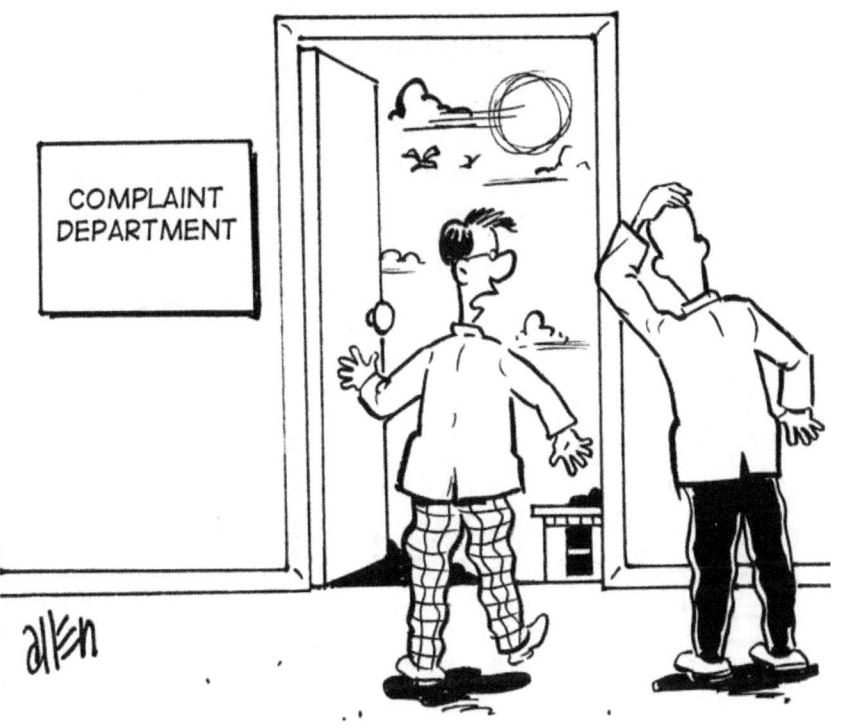

I tried to warn Tia that they don't take
complaints seriously here.

Enter your caption:

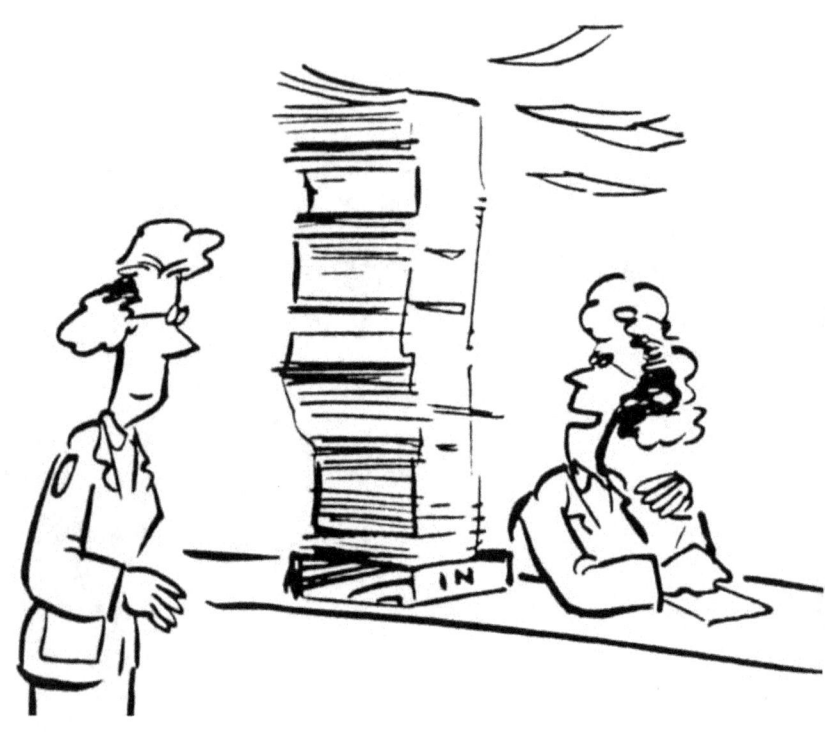

Inbox!!?.....is that what that
thing is?

Enter your caption:

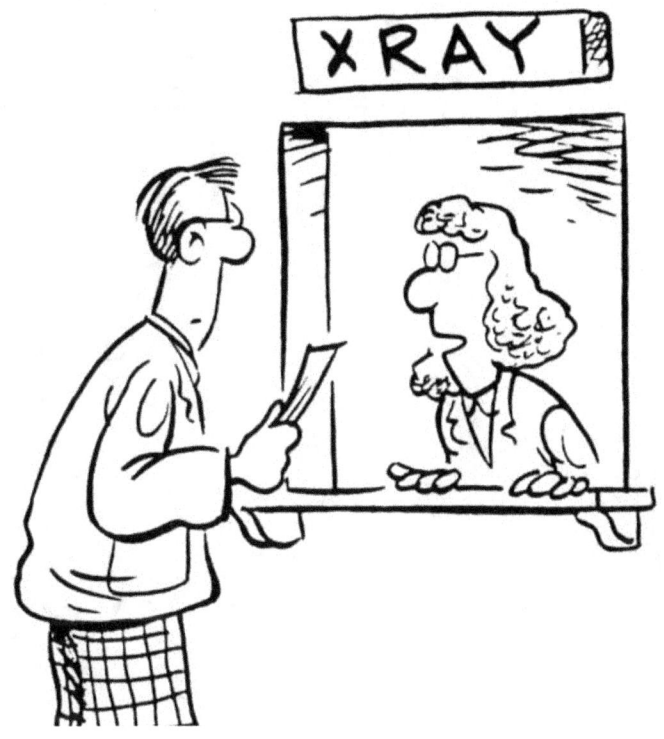

You have got to be kidding! I have Xray vision too!

Enter your caption:

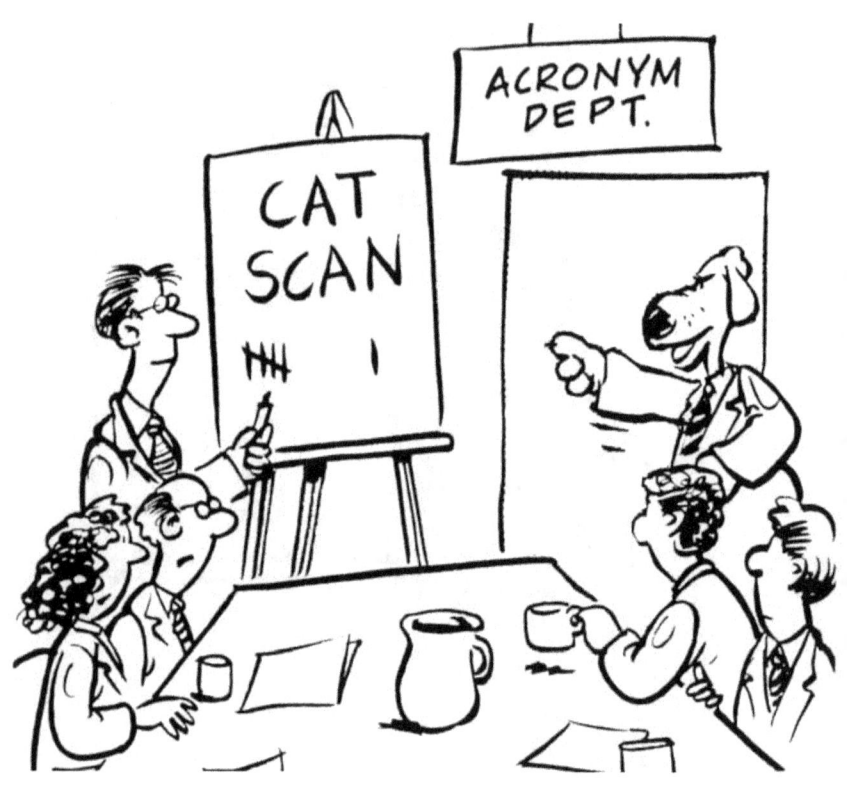

I demand a recount!

Enter your caption:

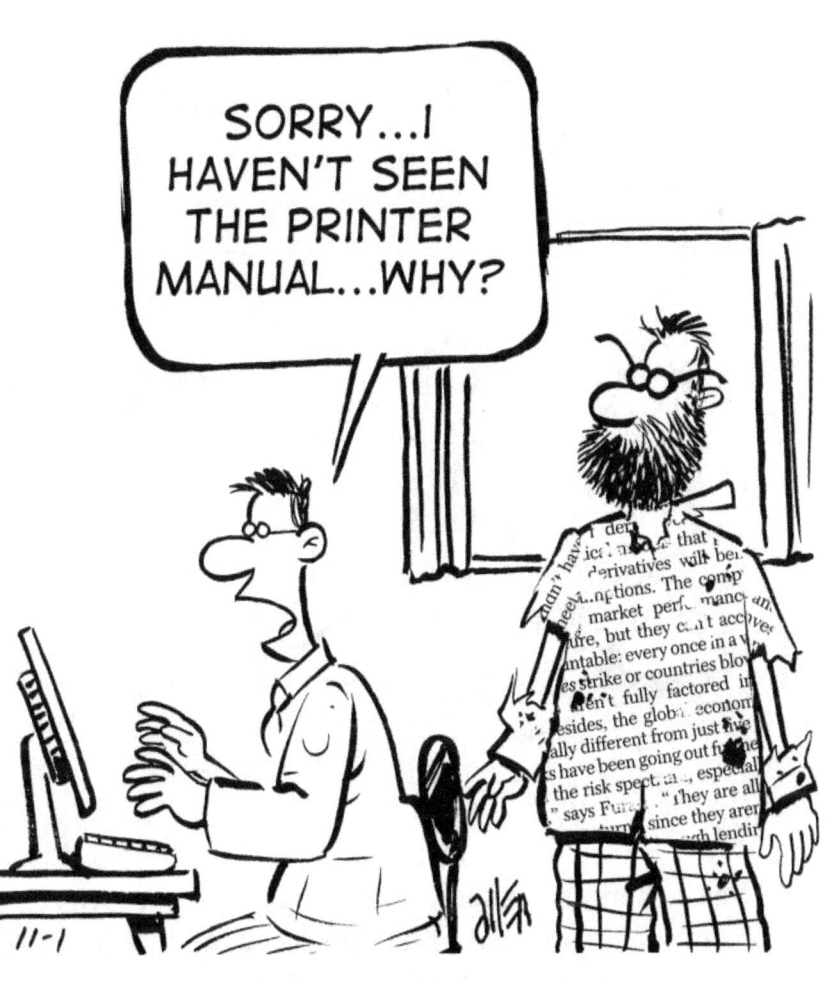

Enter your caption:

_____

_____

_____

_____

_____

_____

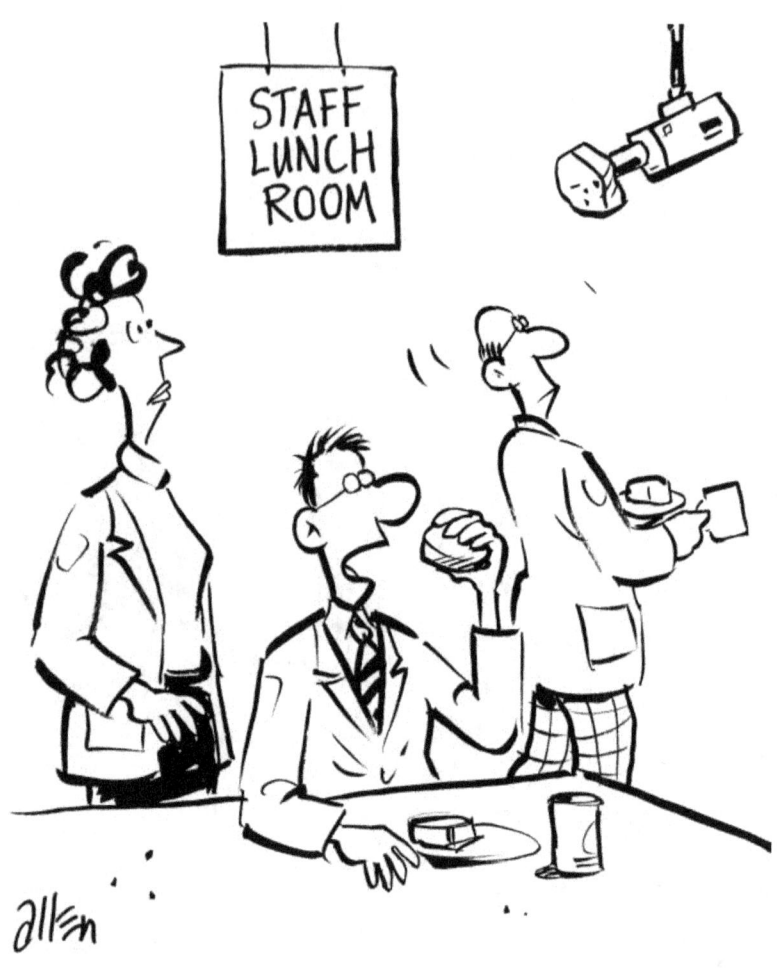

Yes…there is a biscuit on the lens of the security camera! I got tired of having someone looking over my shoulder while I eat.

Enter your caption:

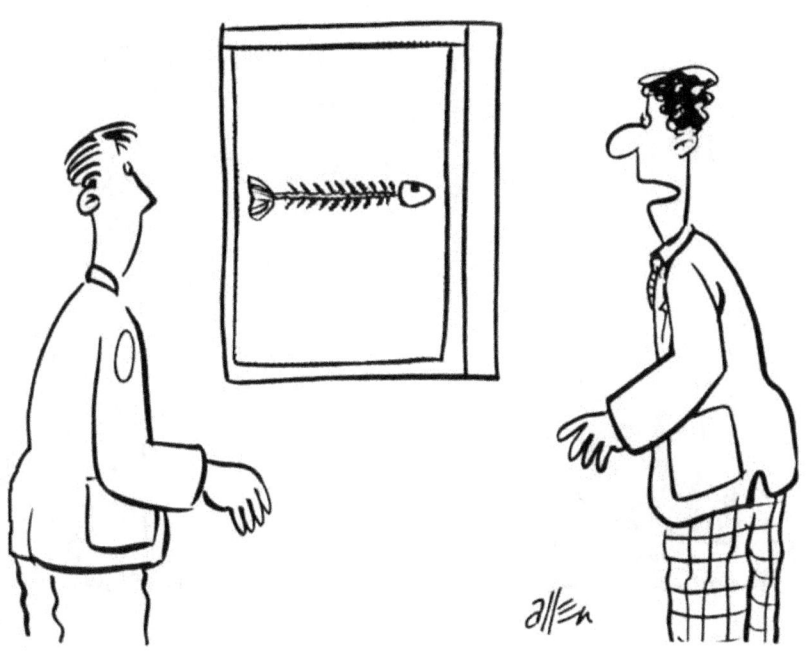

I said I wanted MISTER
Sturgeon's x-ray!

Enter your caption:

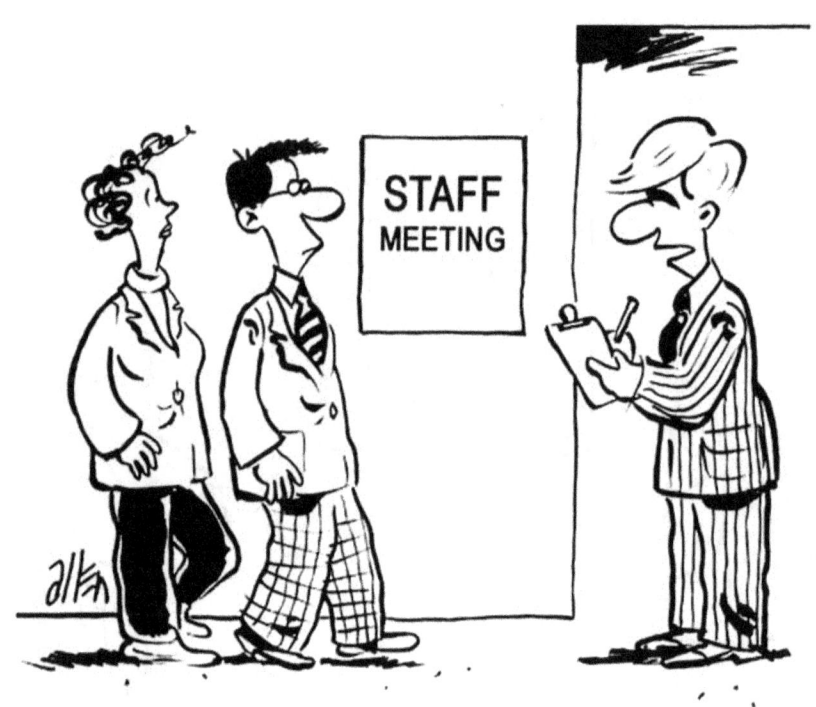

Belly ach'n or non-belly ach'n?

Enter your caption:

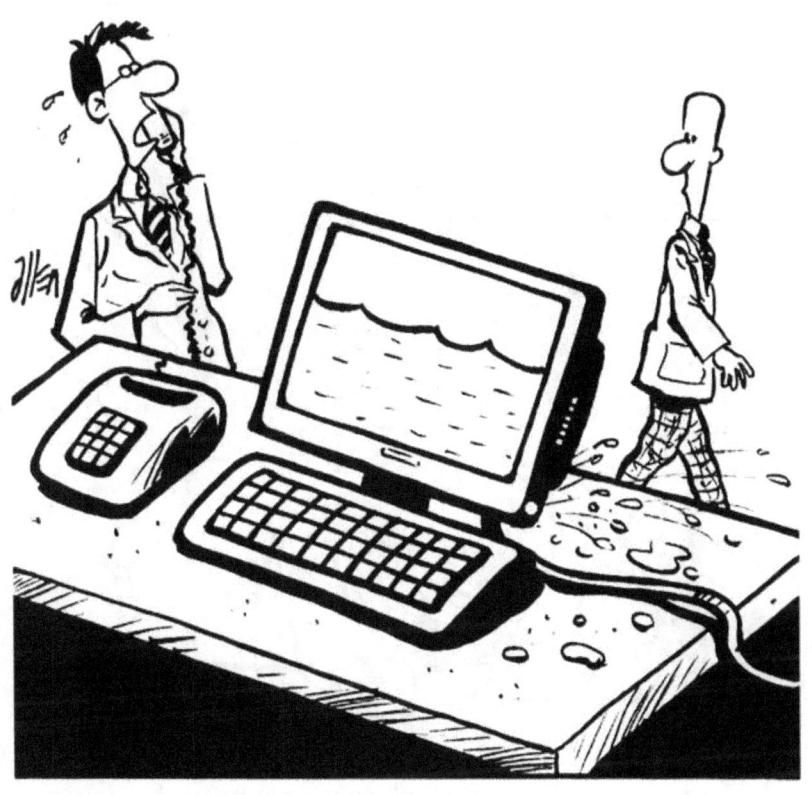

It's not connected to the network...but I think you
connected it to the water line instead!

Enter your caption:

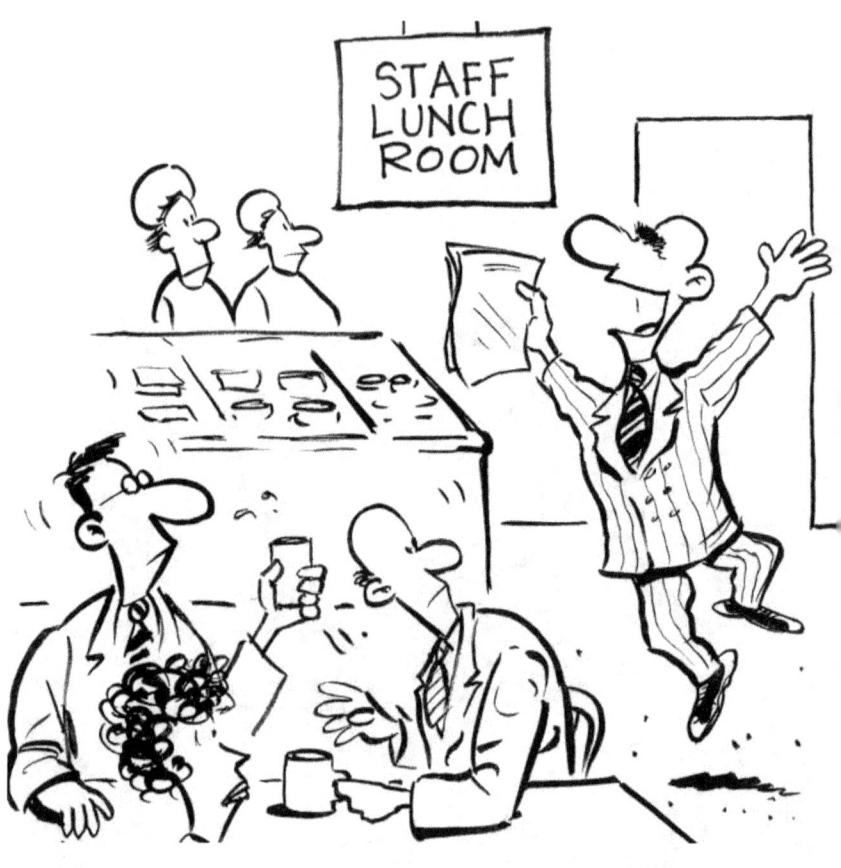

Good news!! The research team came to the same
conclusion that we've had all the time…
"there's no such thing as self-esteem!!"

Enter your caption:

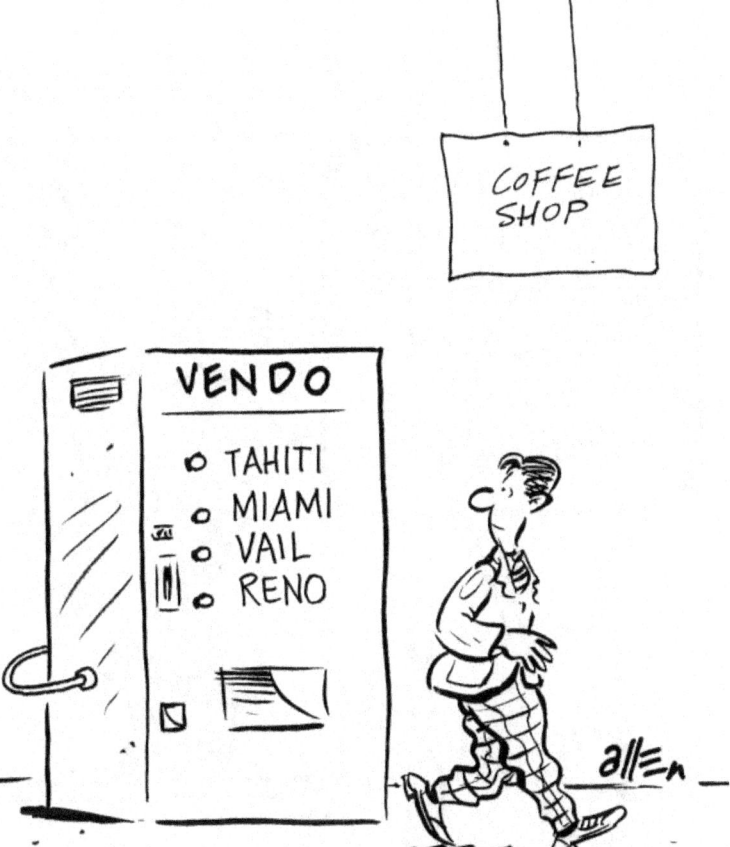

Drat...it doesn't work! I was hoping to get
out of doing this round of treatments.

Enter your caption:

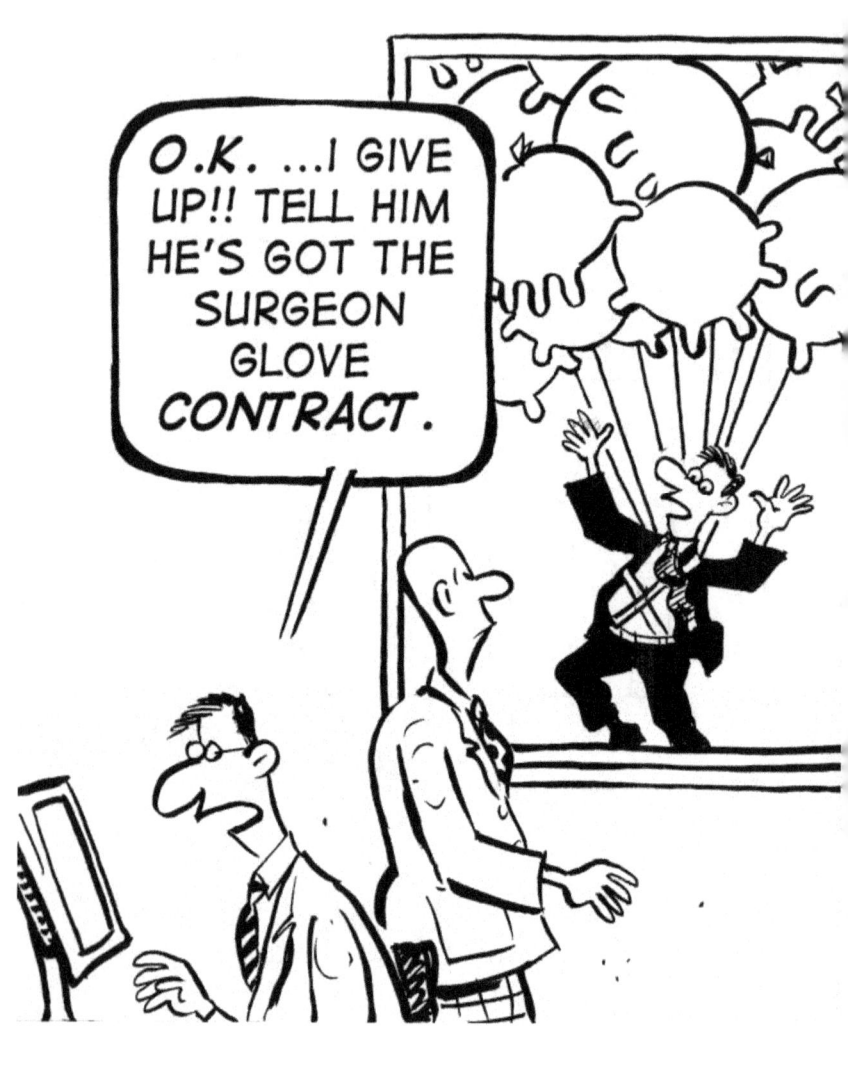

Enter your caption:

_____

_____

_____

_____

_____

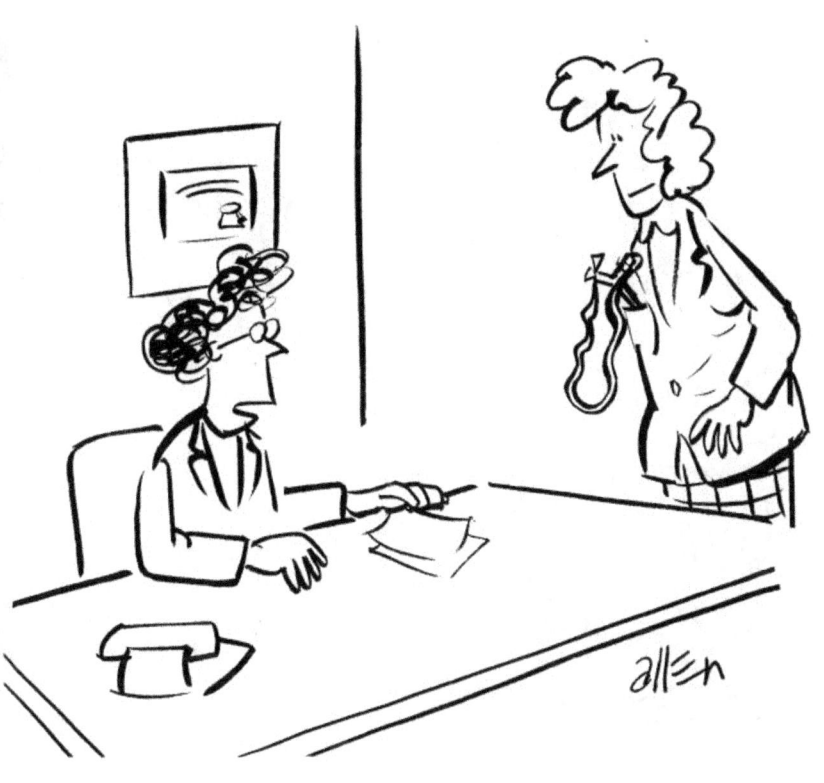

I have an anger management class
too...may I borrow your slingshot?

Enter your caption:

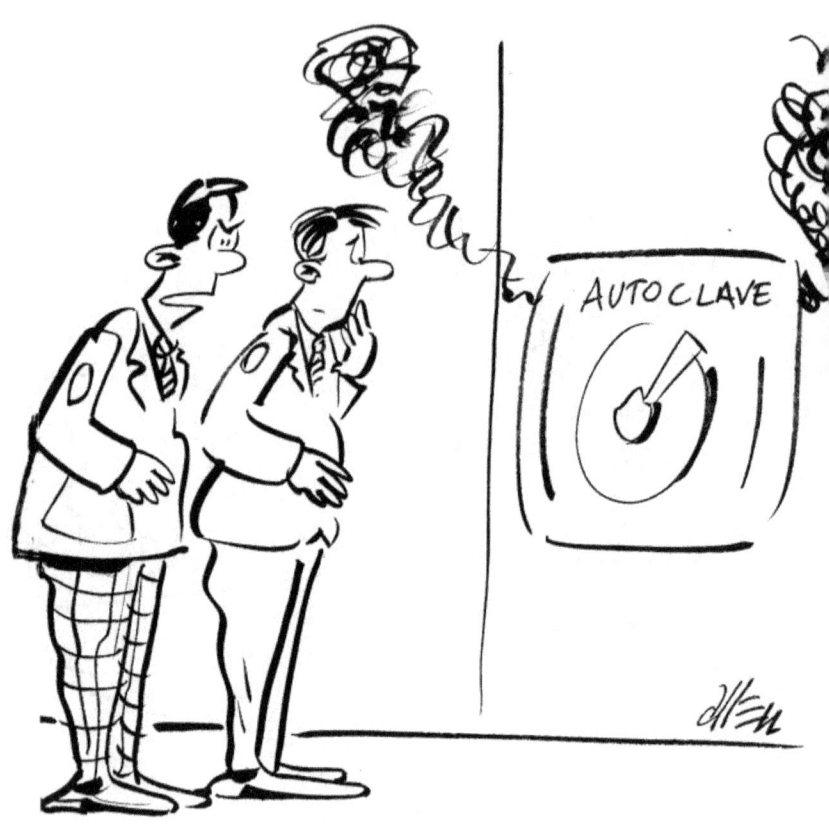

Leslie was so livid about the new schedule...by the way, have you seen it?

Enter your caption:

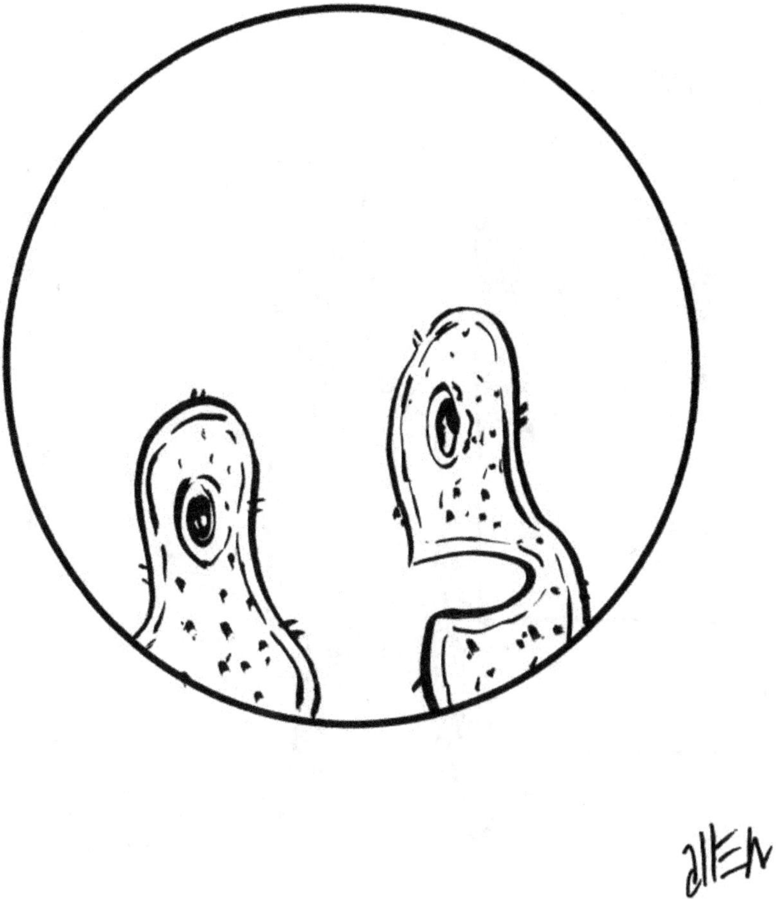

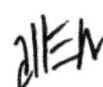

I see it too…it looks like an eye!

Enter your caption:

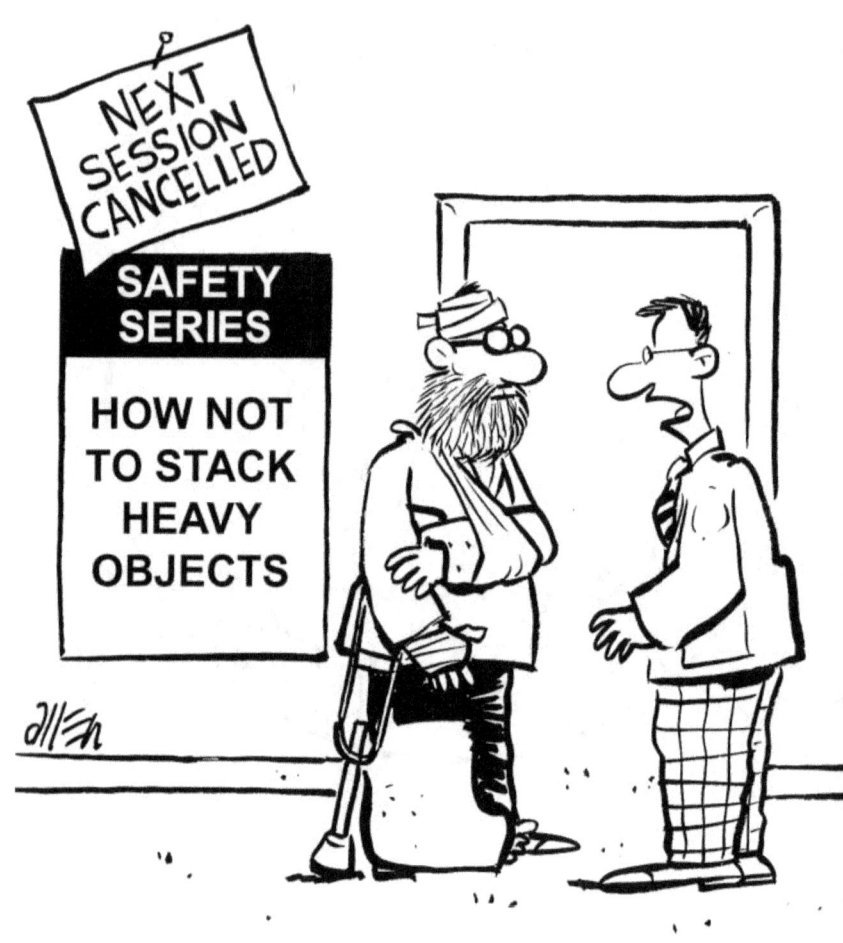

Maybe you should try another
approach.

Enter your caption:

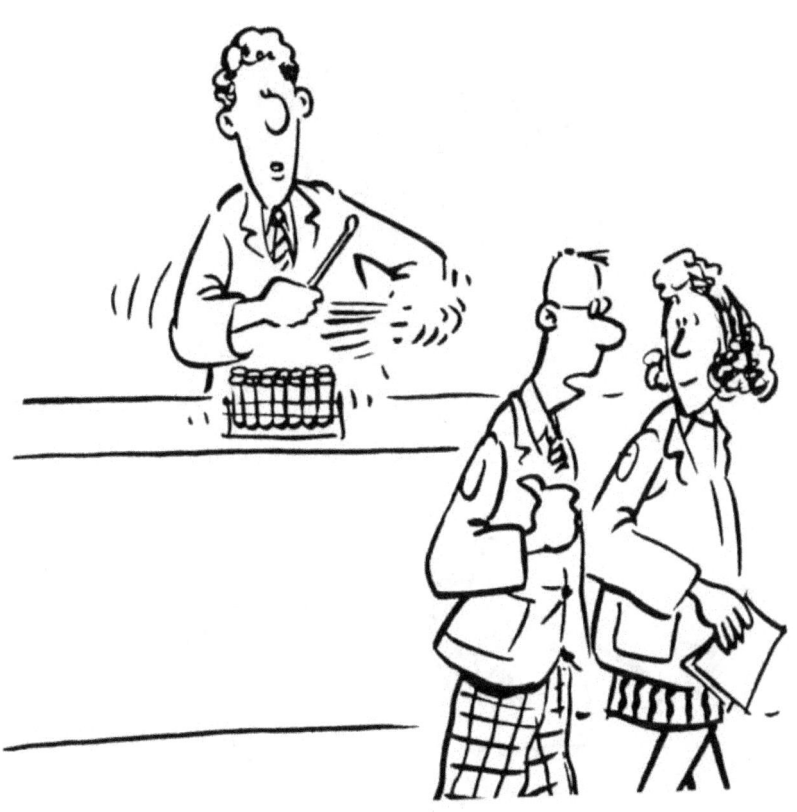

I think Kevin has too much time on his hands...
he's playing "flight of the bumble bee" on
the test tubes.

Enter your caption:

_____

_____

_____

_____

_____

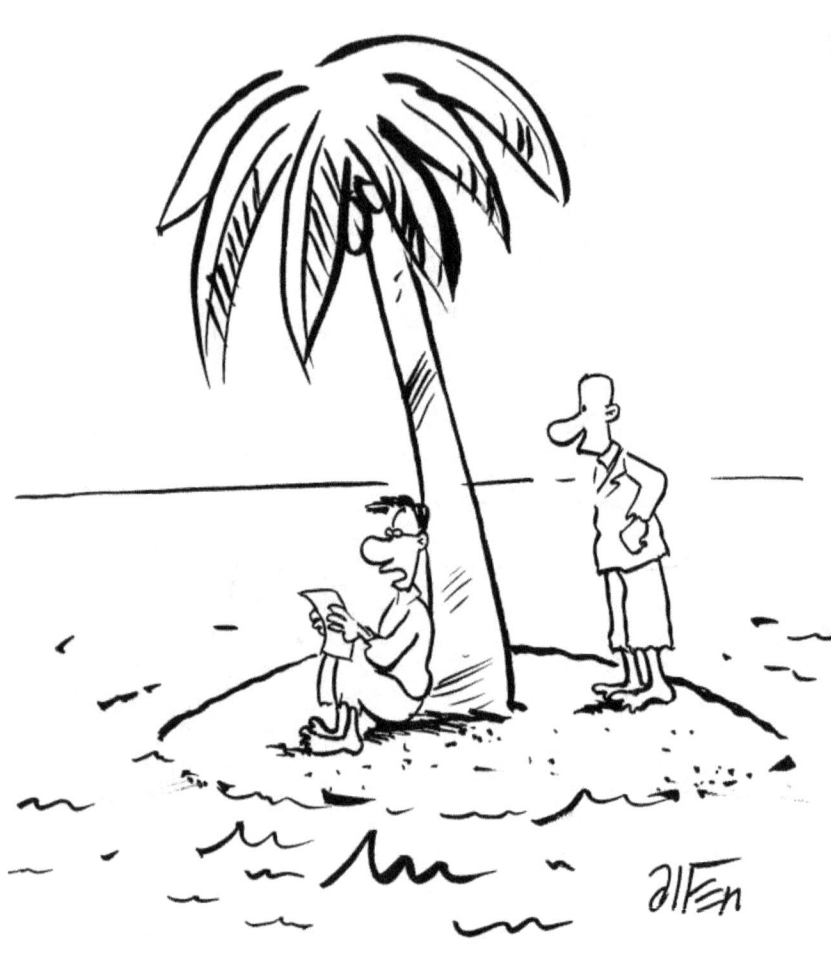

Just what do you mean by
EMINENT DOMAIN!?!!

Enter your caption:

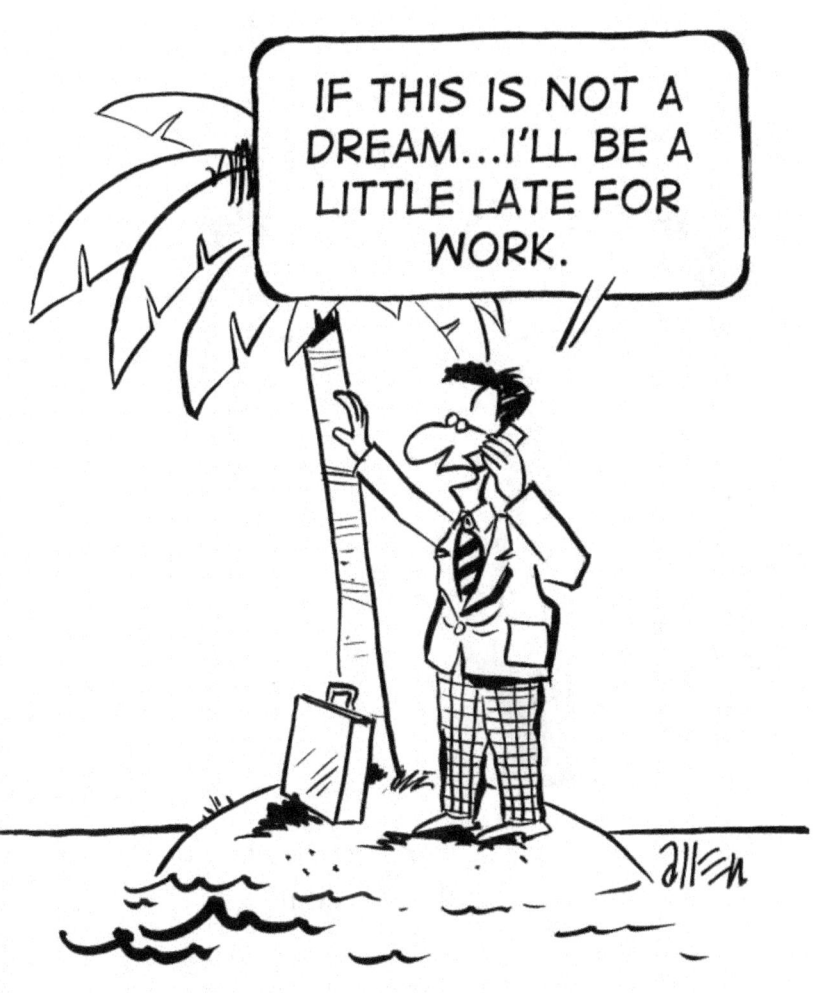

Enter your caption:

_____

_____

_____

_____

_____

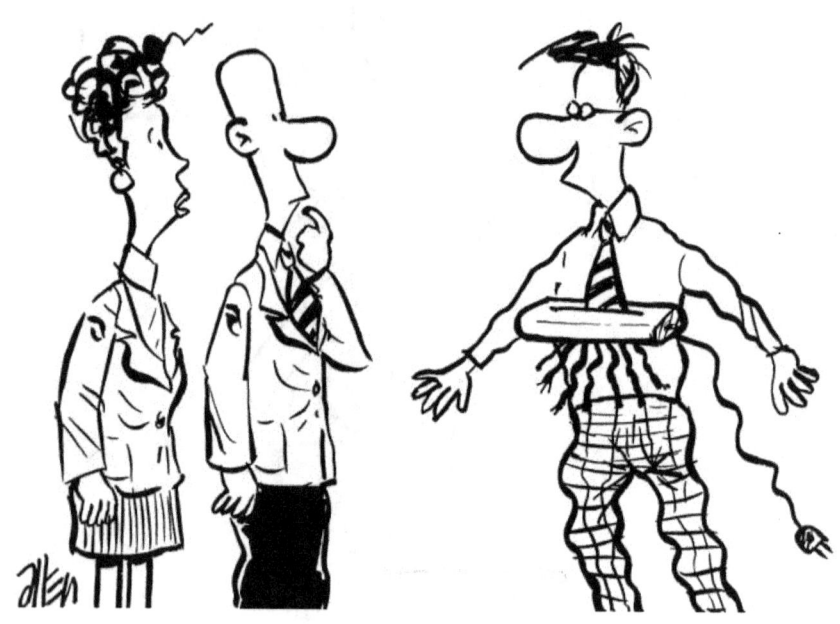

I hope you have a good excuse why you didn't
finish the shredding.

Enter your caption:

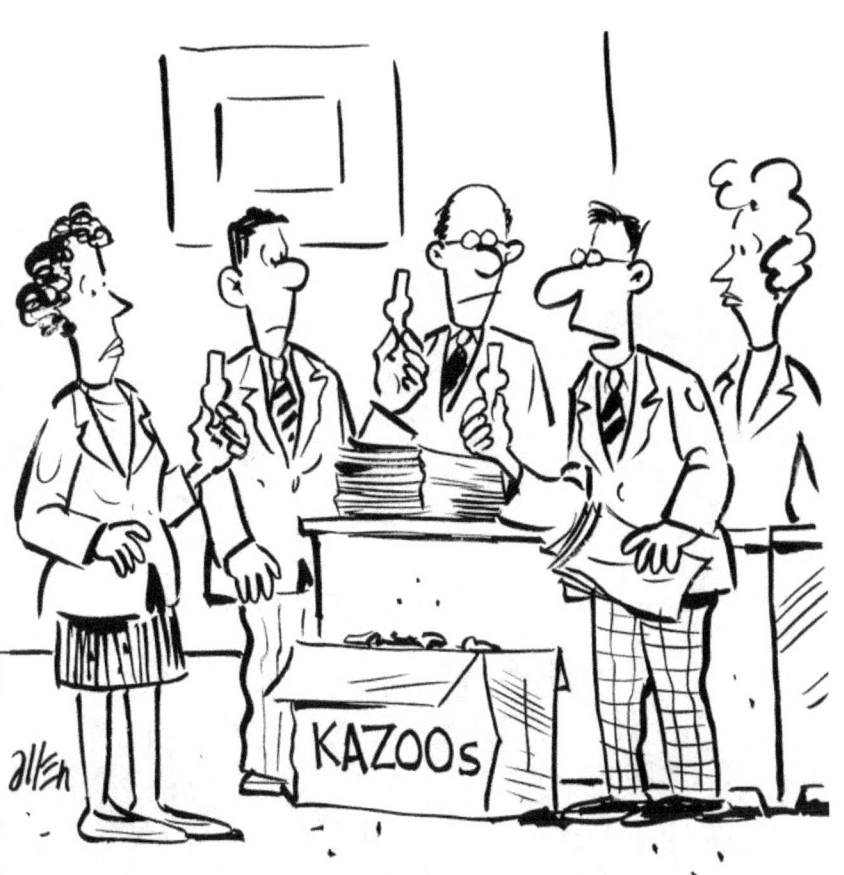

Before we go over the new budget figures…I thought we would start with an up-beat tune called "I feel good."

Enter your caption:

_____

_____

_____

_____

_____

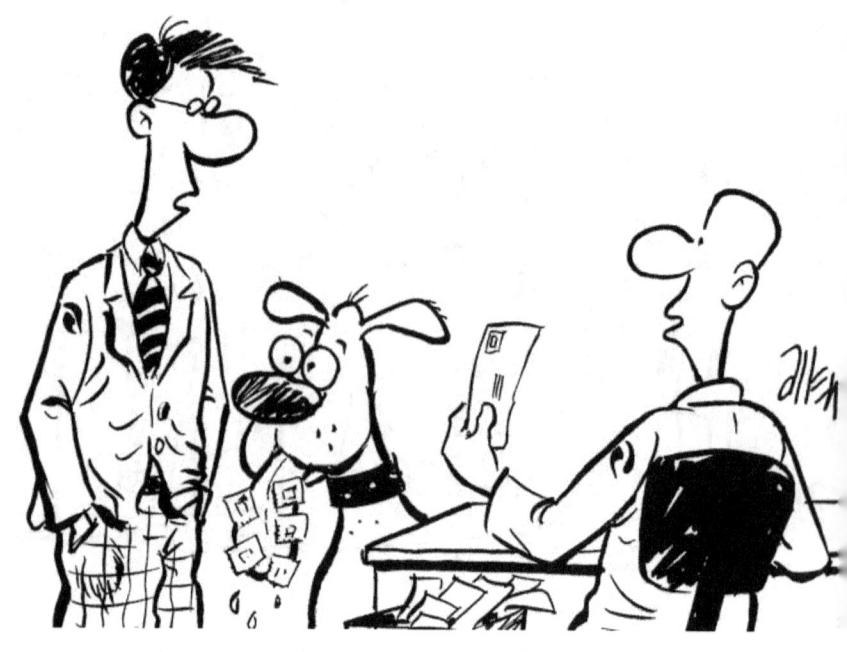

Dog…Schmog! This is a mean
stamp-licking machine!

Enter your caption:

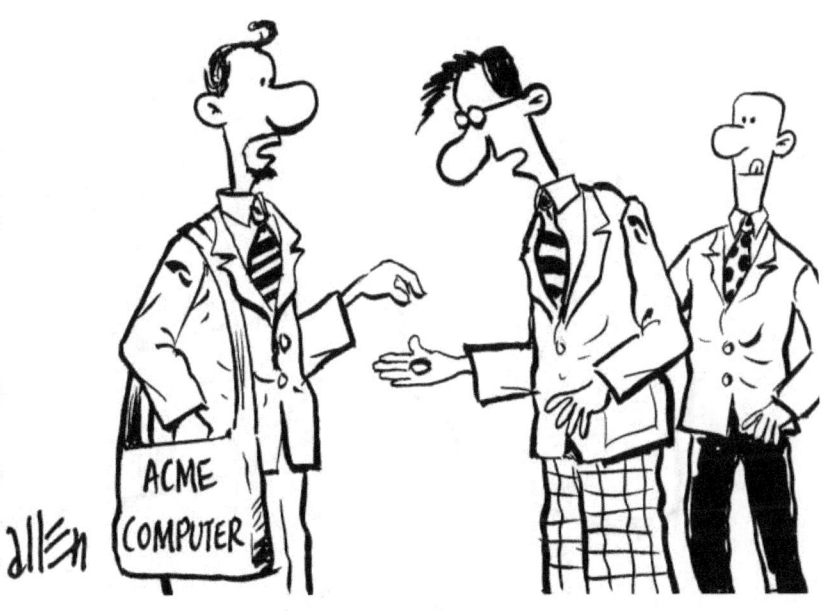

I know they're getting smaller but...that's
not a computer! That's a milk dud!

Enter your caption:

_____

_____

_____

_____

_____

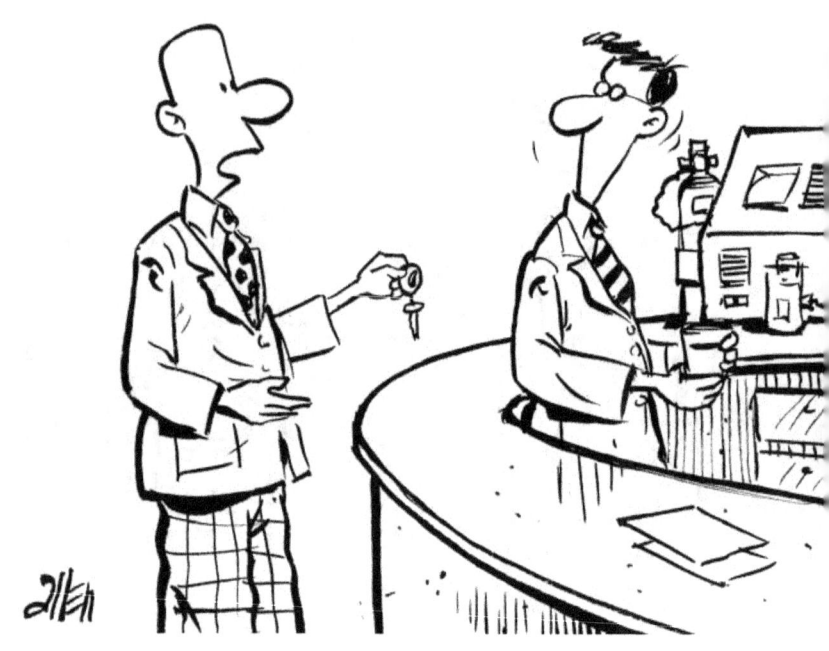

...the good news is I found your steering wheel.

Enter your caption:

_____

_____

_____

_____

_____

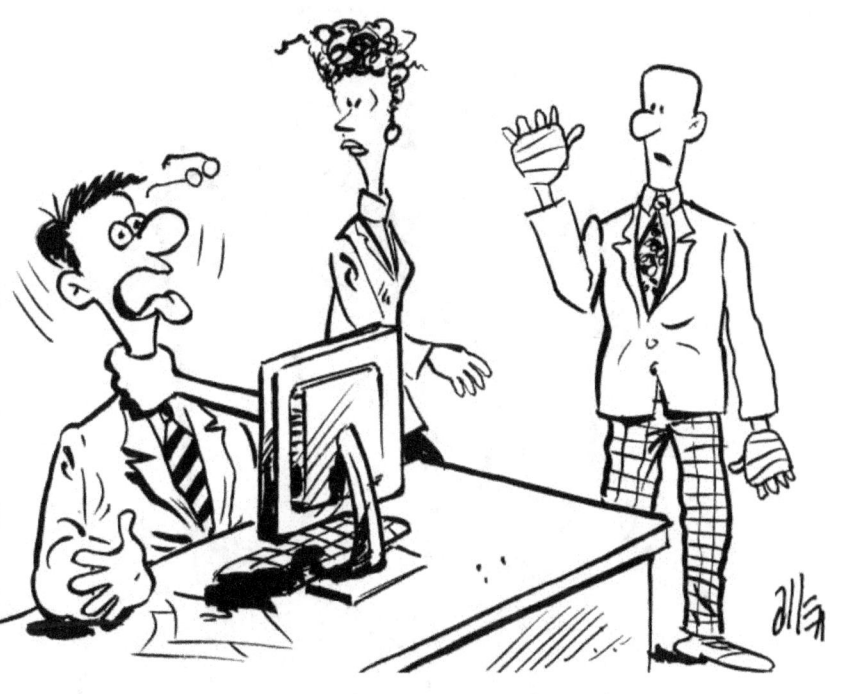

That new software program is unforgiving! It
broke both of my hands.

Enter your caption:

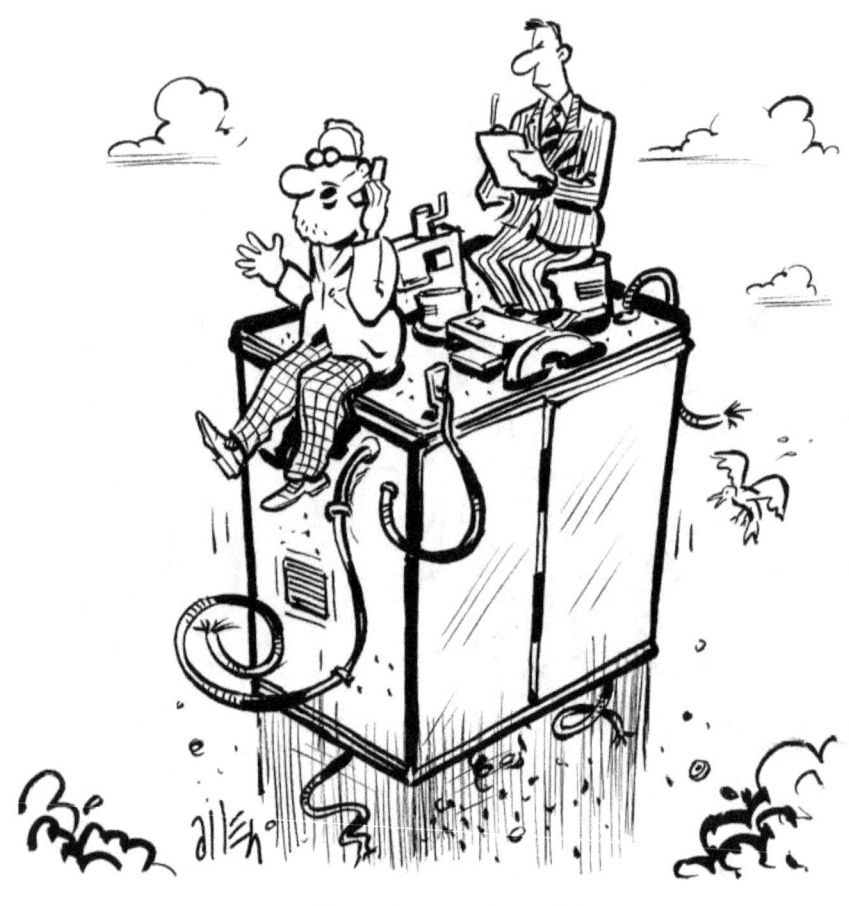

I'll explain it later…the five north elevator
didn't pass the inspection.

Enter your caption:

_____

_____

_____

_____

_____

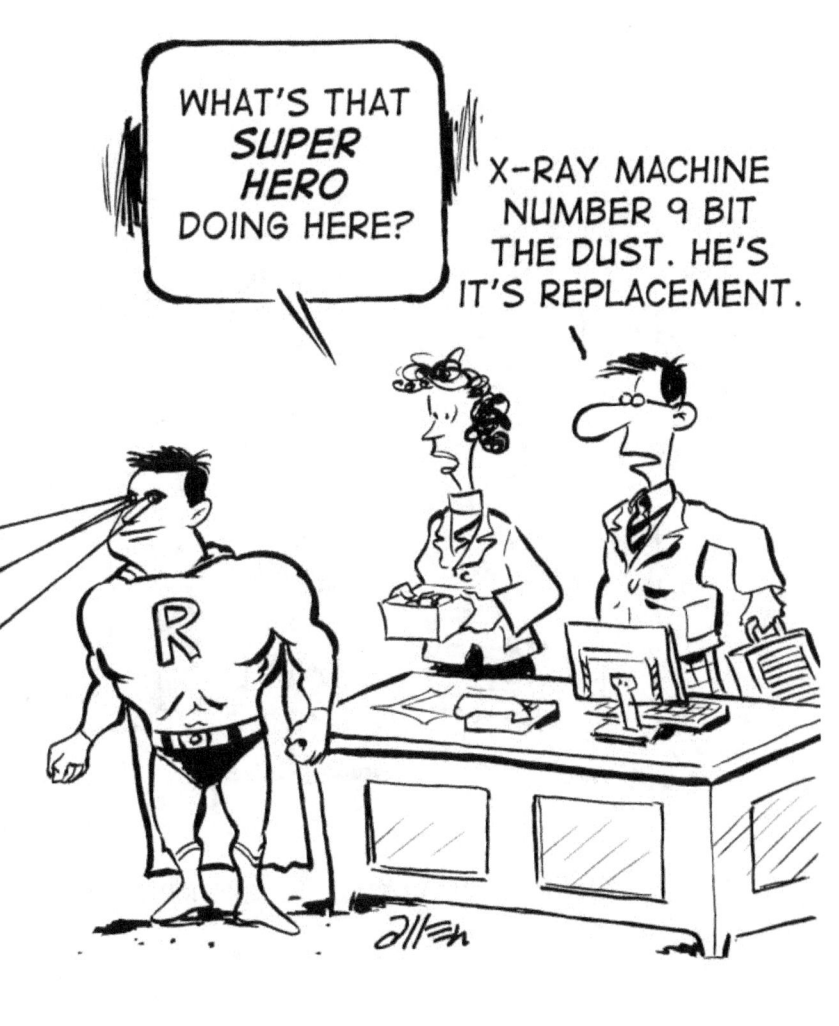

Enter your caption:

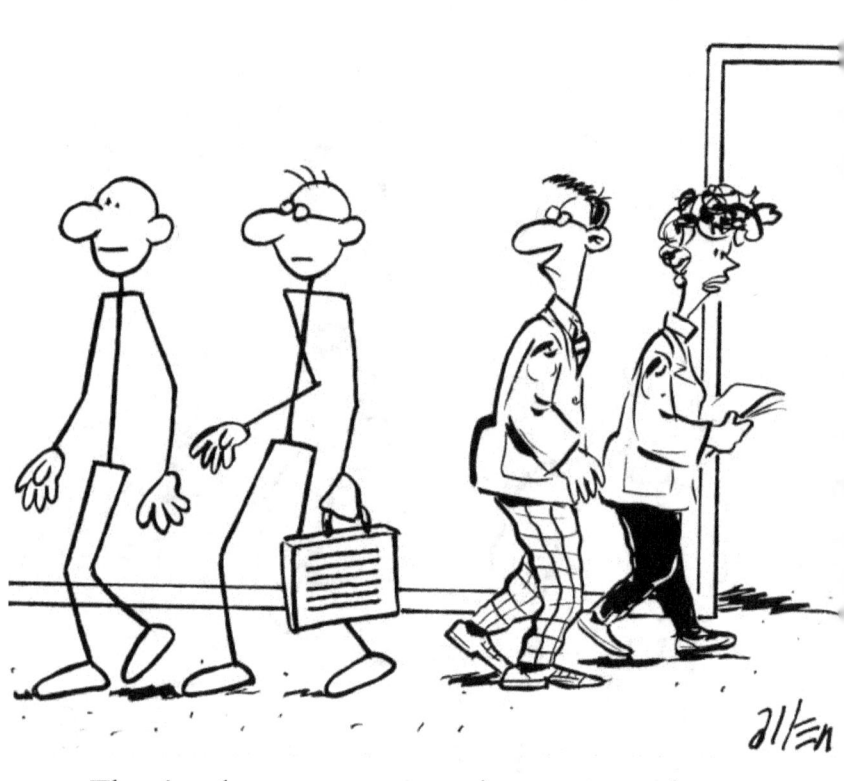

They're the new cost containment consultants.

Enter your caption:

_____

_____

_____

_____

_____

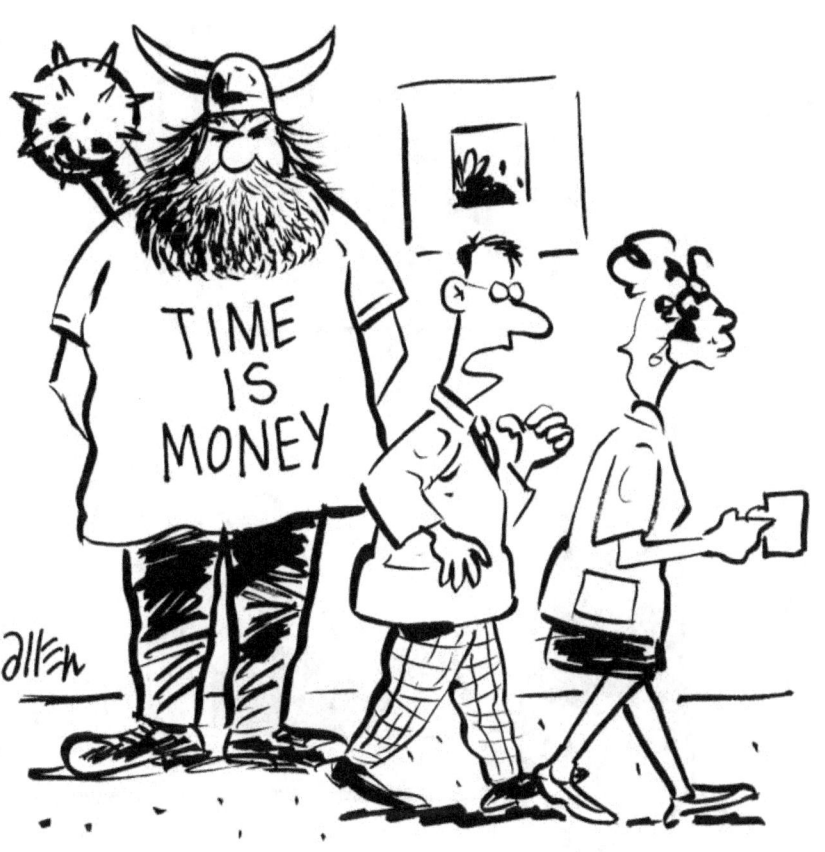

That's the new accountant.

Enter your caption:

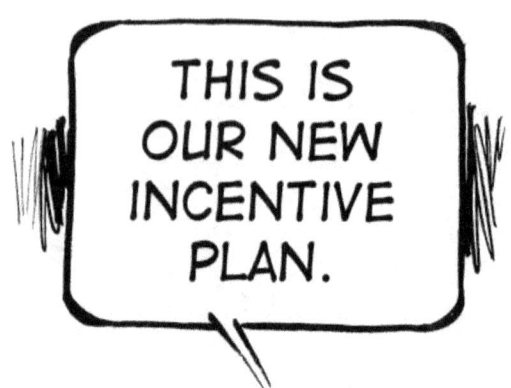

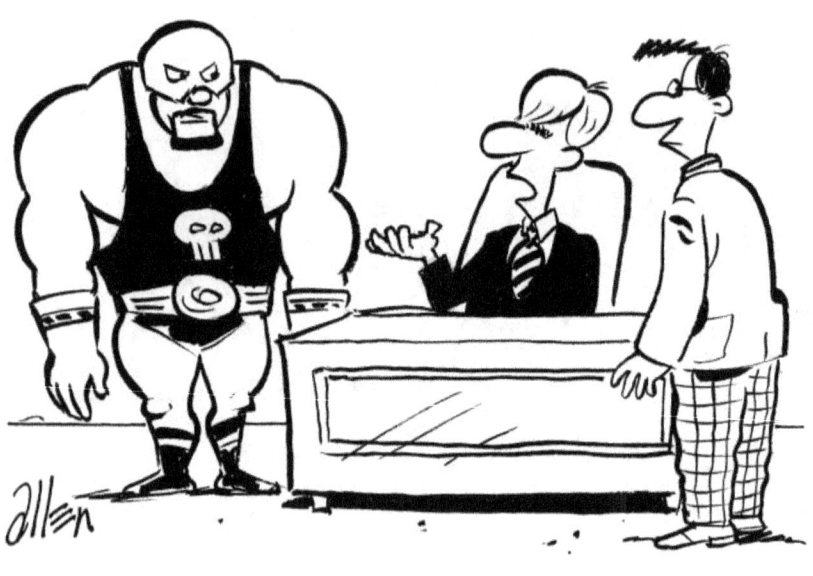

Enter your caption:

_____

_____

_____

_____

_____

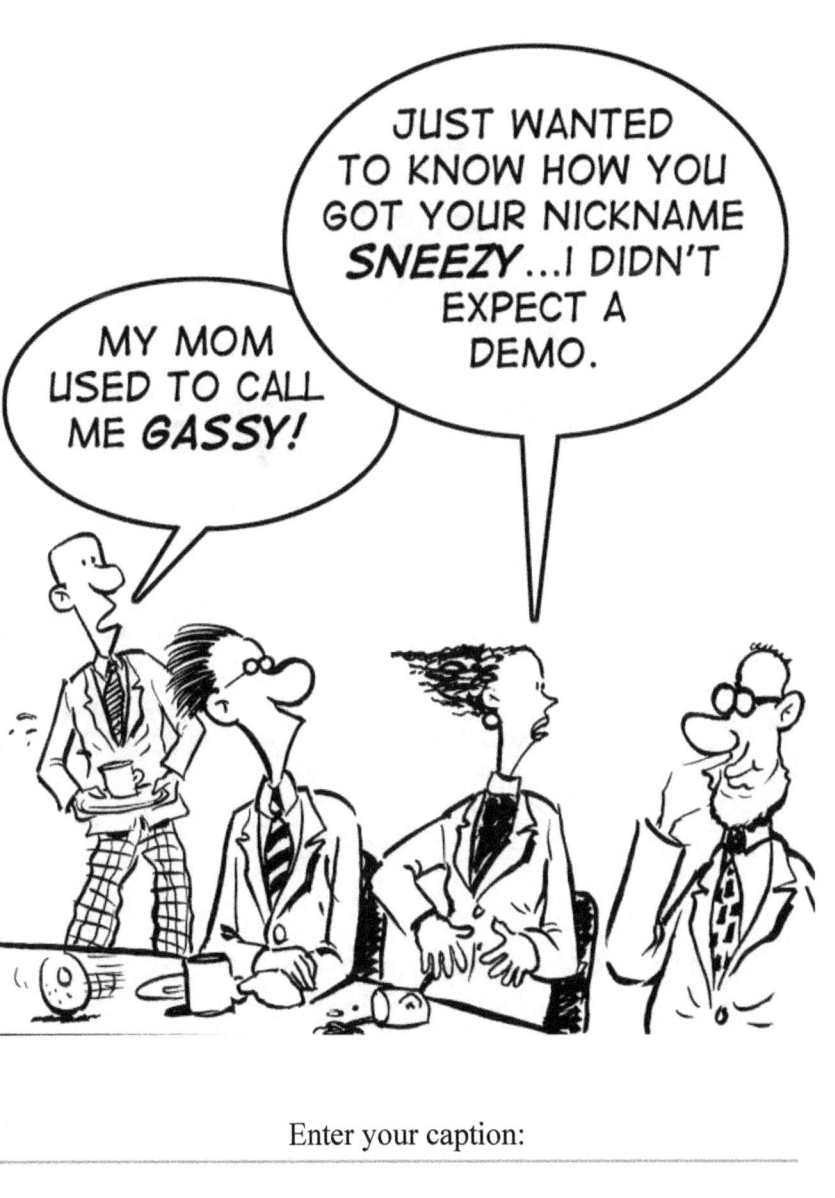

Enter your caption:

_____

_____

_____

_____

_____

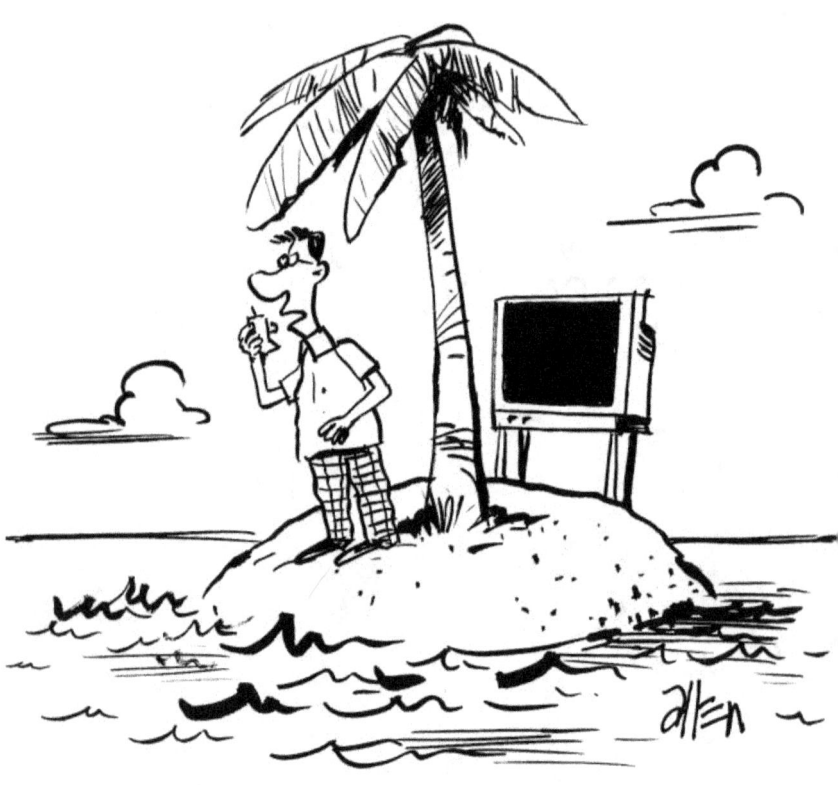

I called in to tell them I couldn't make it and they said I just won the best all time excuse for calling in for work.

Enter your caption:

_____

_____

_____

_____

_____

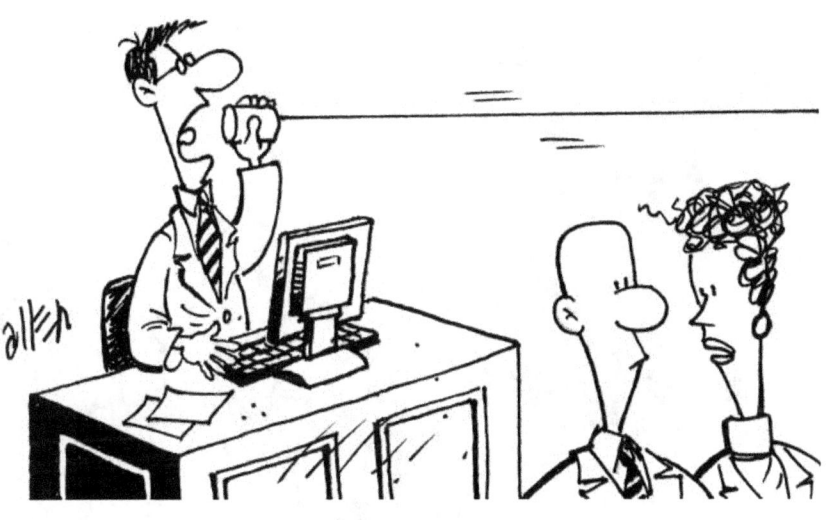

They gave him $7,000 for that cost-cutting
suggestion.

Enter your caption:

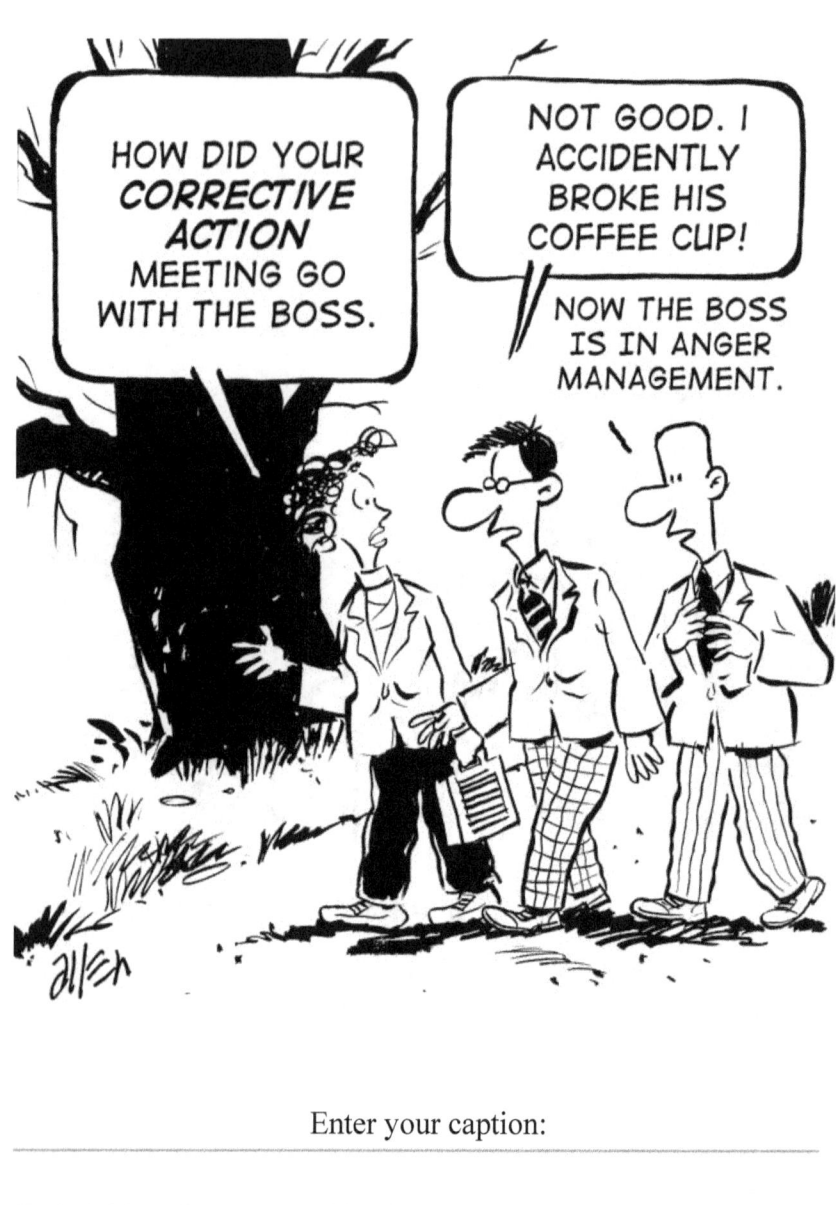

Enter your caption:

_____

_____

_____

_____

_____

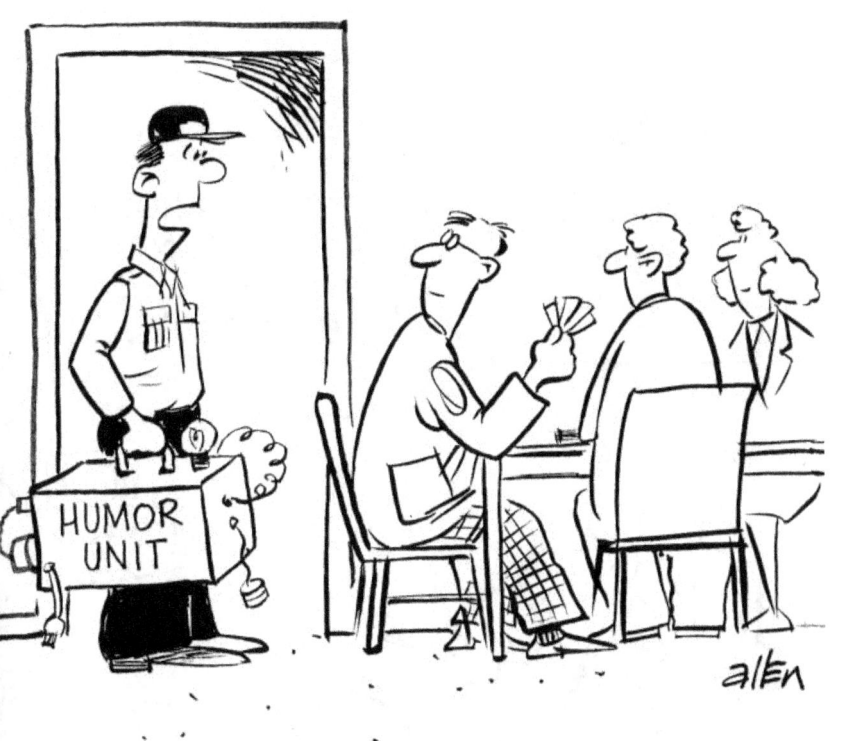

I got here as soon as I could....I heard things
were a little too normal in your department.

Enter your caption:

_____

_____

_____

_____

_____

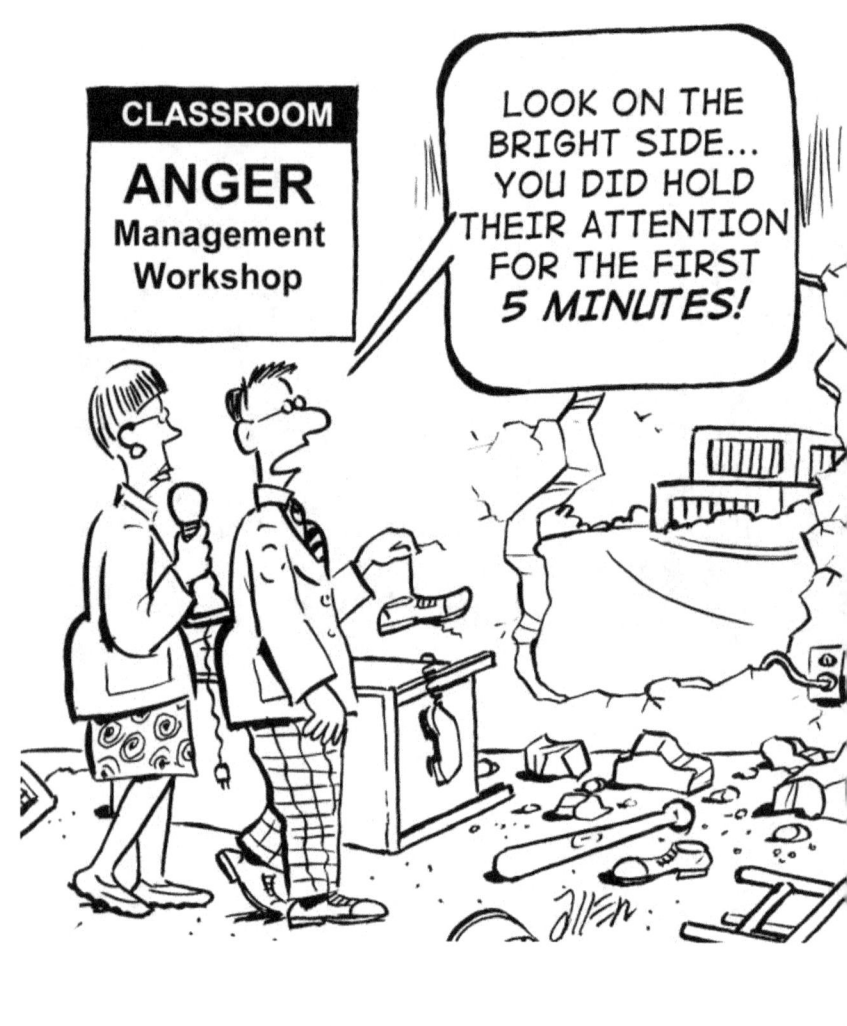

Enter your caption:

_____

_____

_____

_____

_____

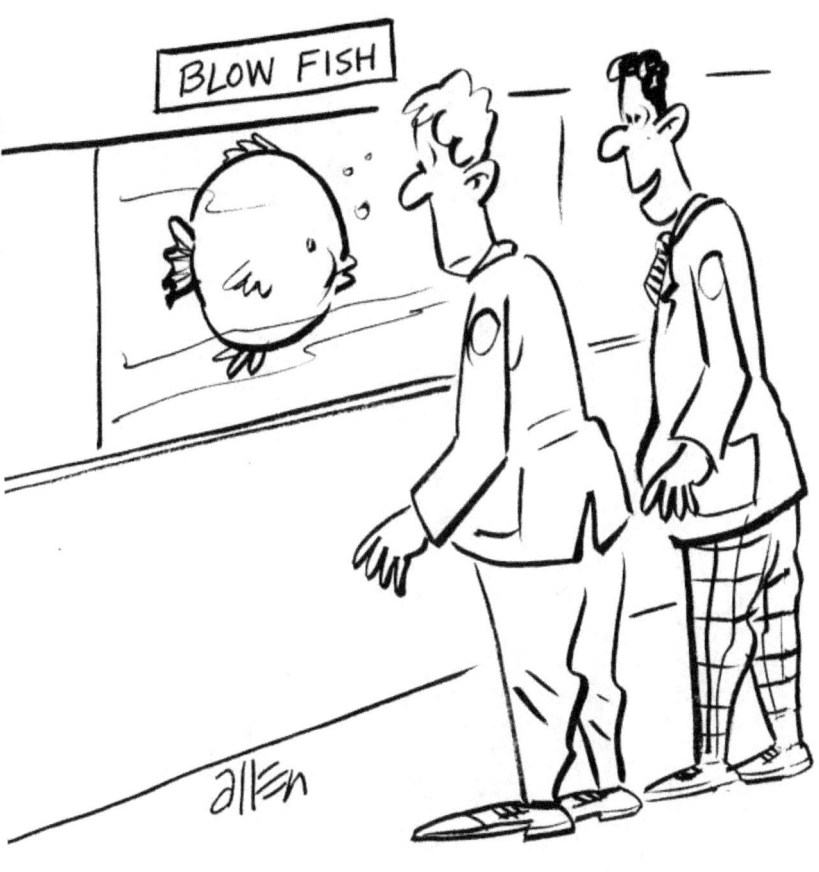

1.2 liters...no way! I'd say it's more like 3.5 liters for it's vital capacity.

Enter your caption:

_____

_____

_____

_____

_____

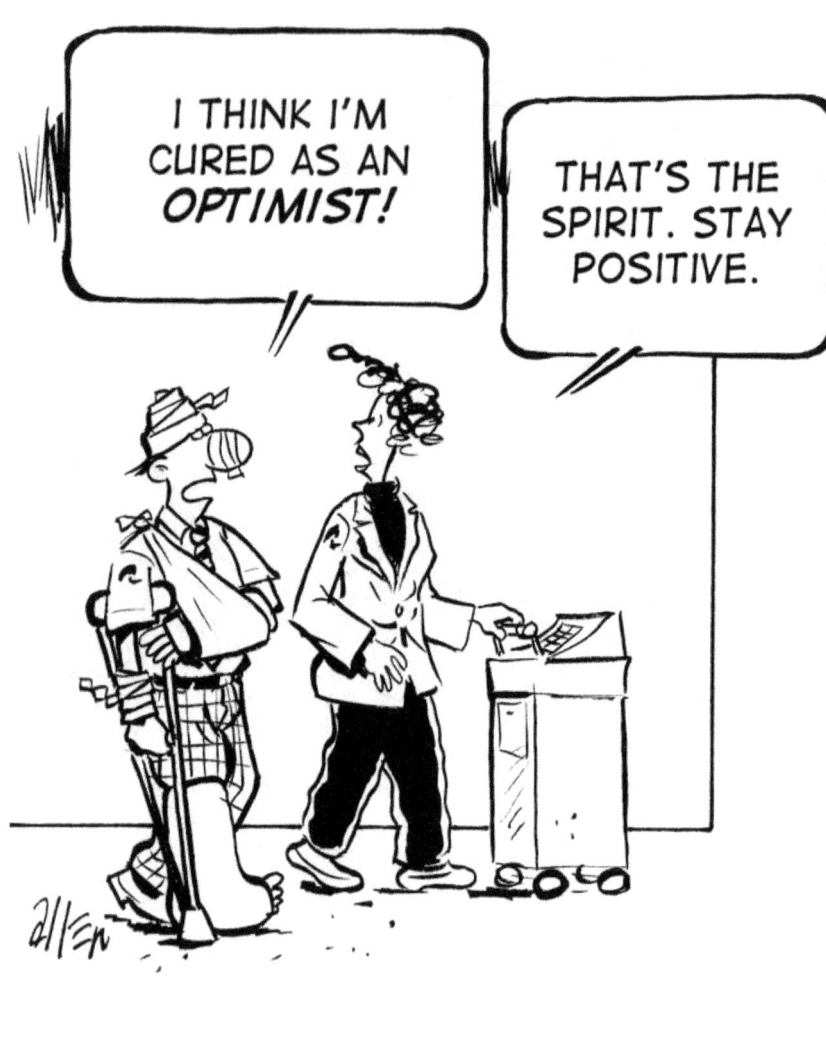

Enter your caption:

_____

_____

_____

_____

_____

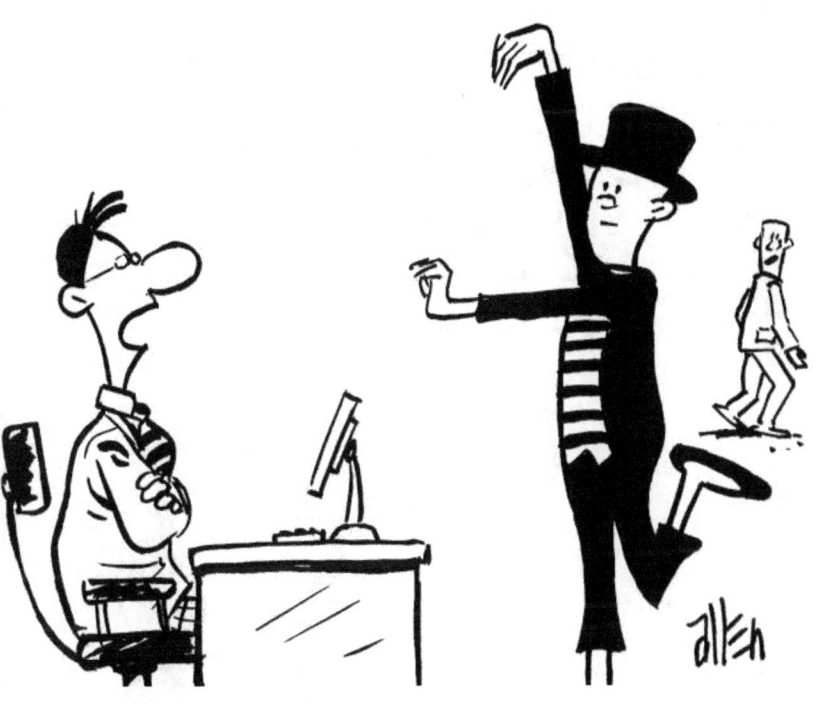

What do you mean the staffing agency ran out of
therapists and only have mimes left?

Enter your caption:

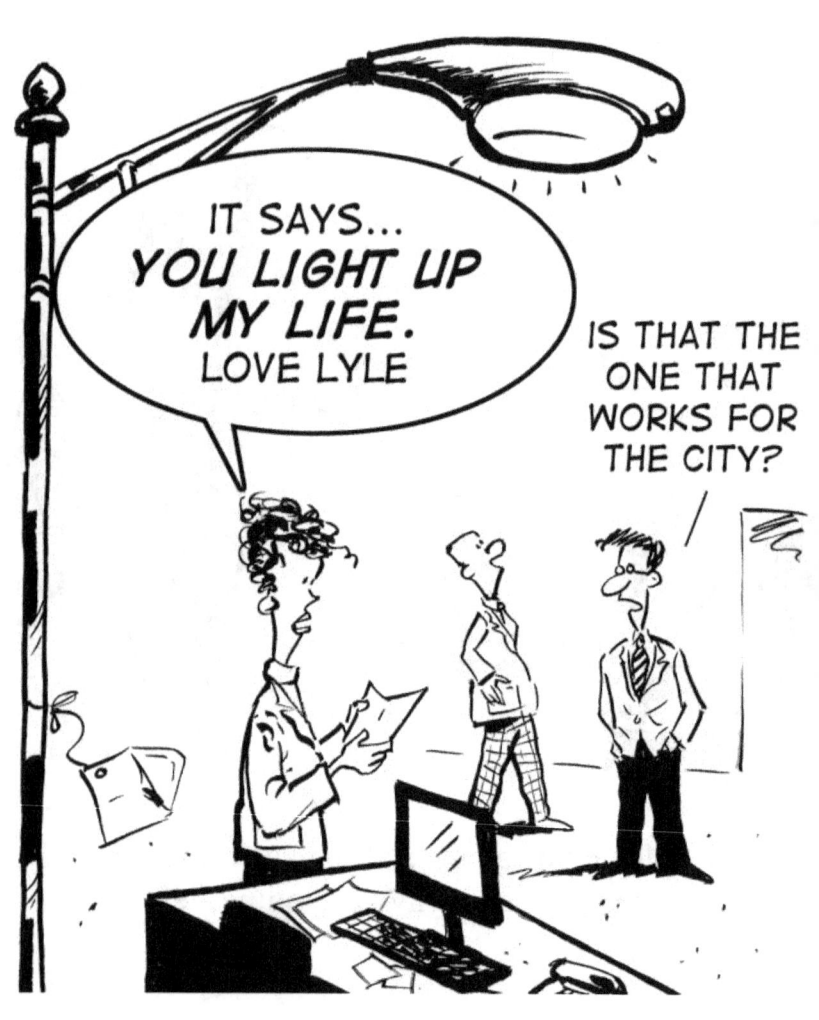

Enter your caption:

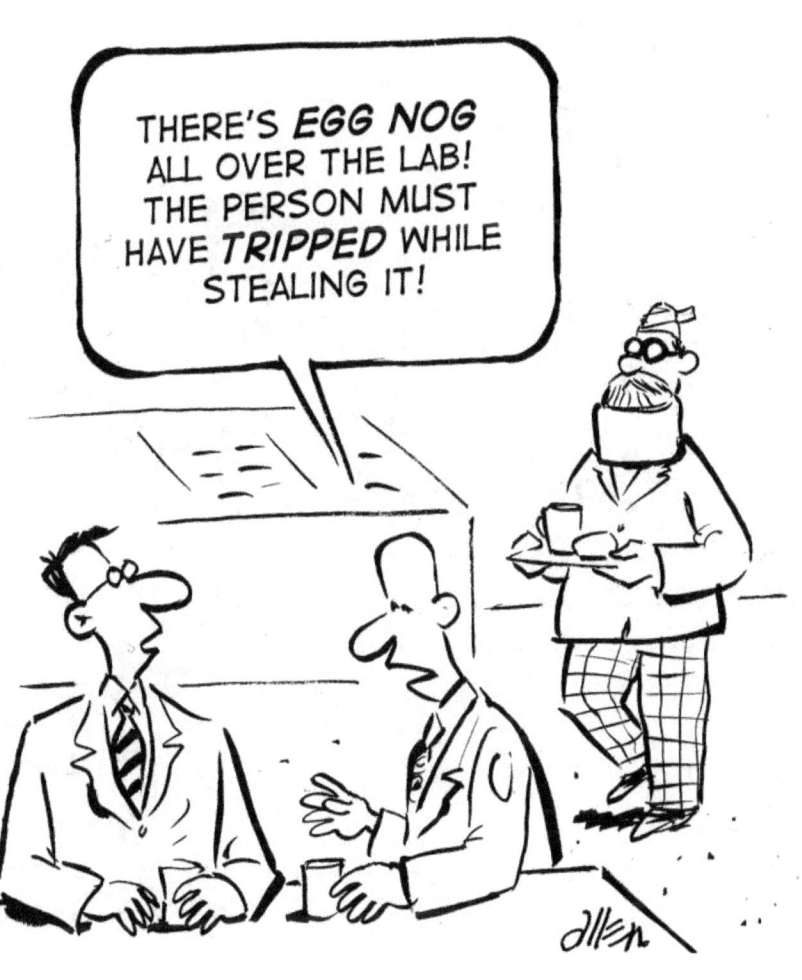

Enter your caption:

_____

_____

_____

_____

_____

_____

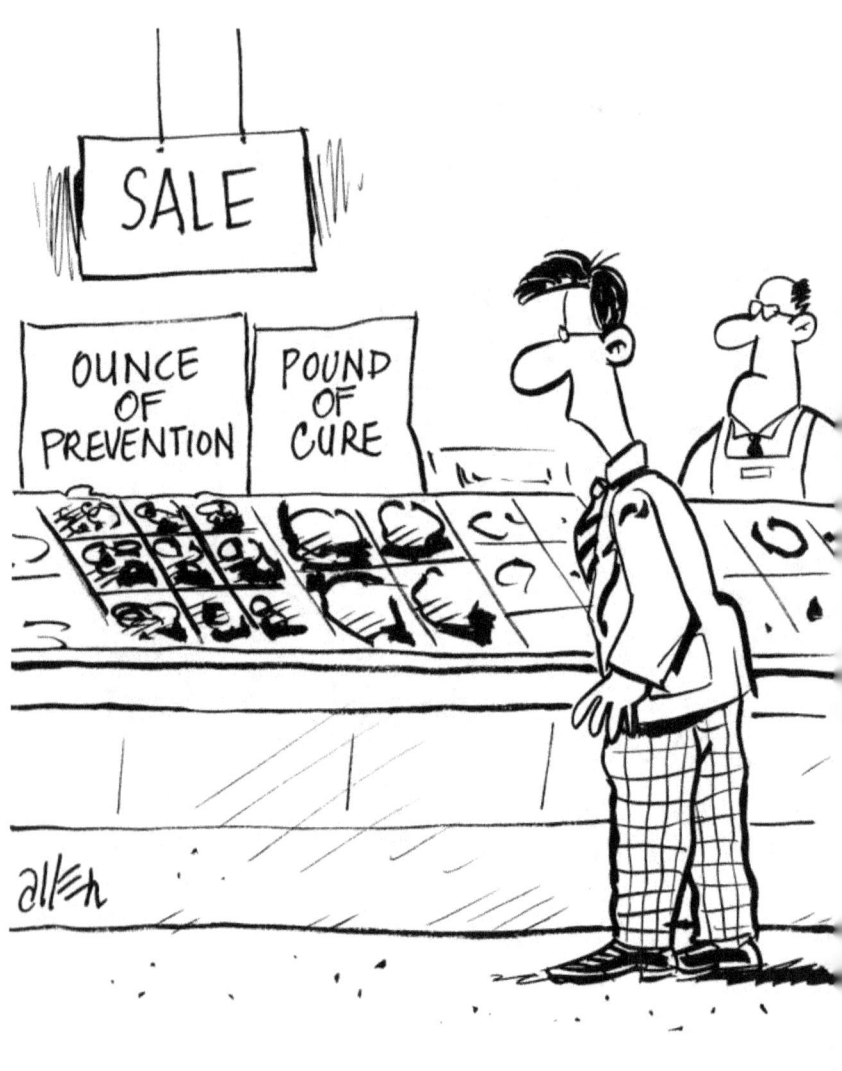

Enter your caption:

_____

_____

_____

_____

_____

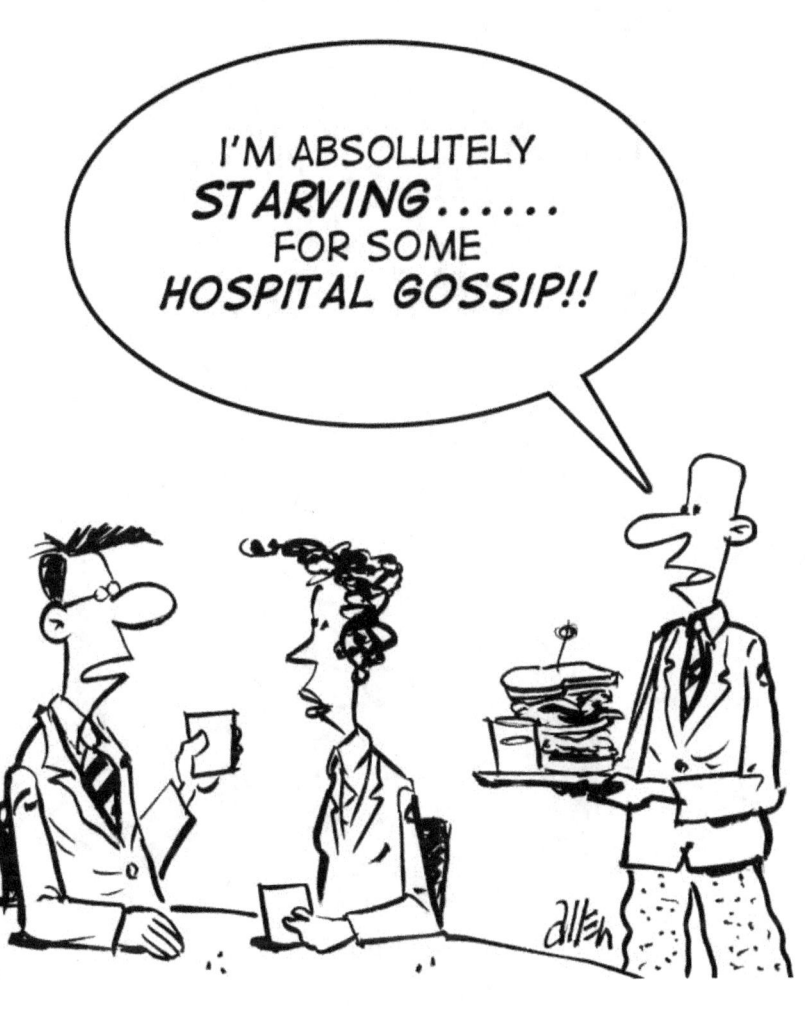

Enter your caption:

_____

_____

_____

_____

_____

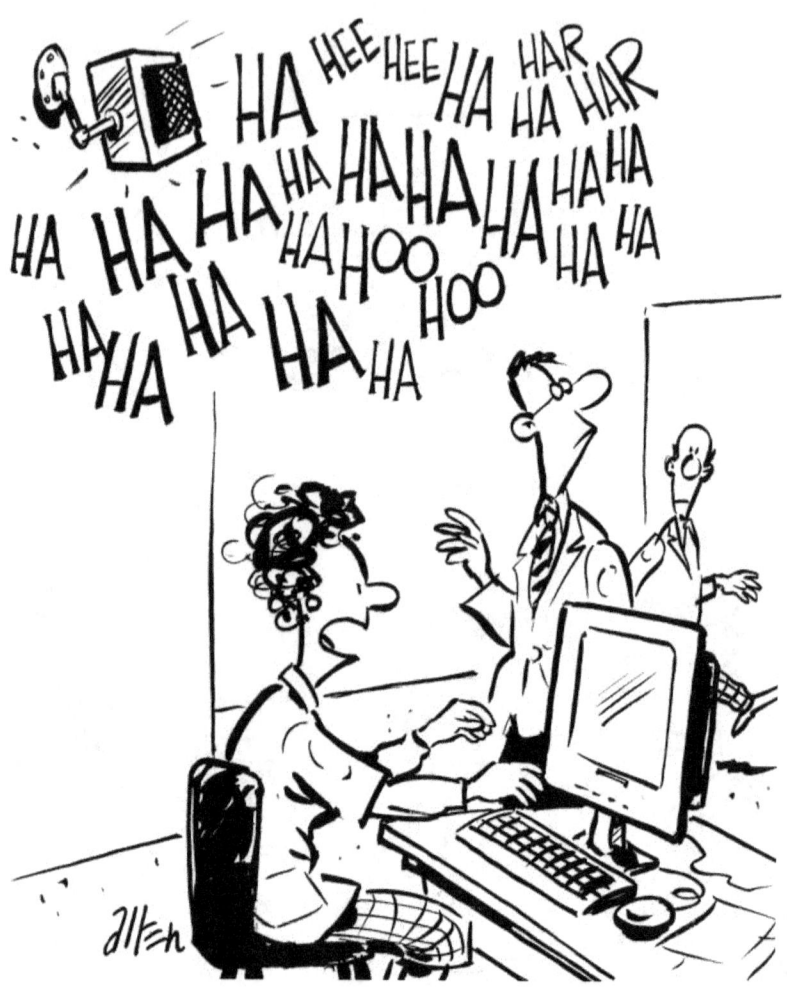

I'm tired of nobody getting my jokes…so I had a laugh track installed.

Enter your caption:

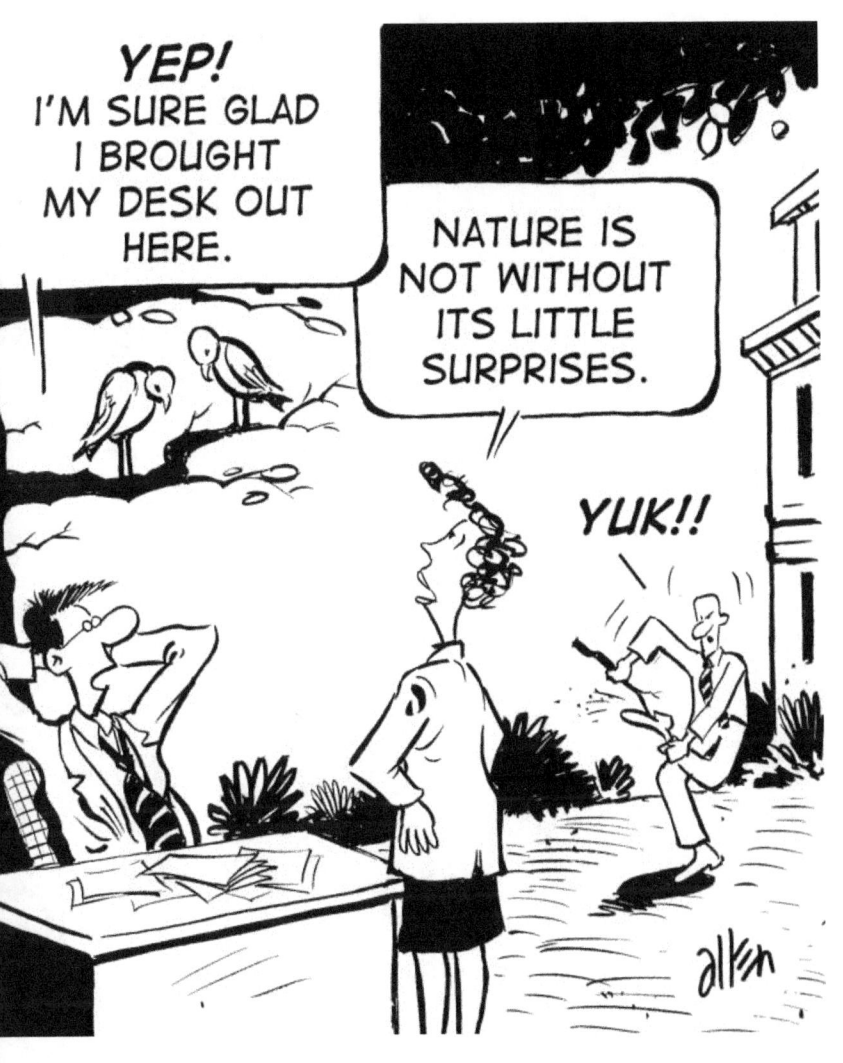

Enter your caption:

_____

_____

_____

_____

_____